RECENT ADVANCES IN DERMATO-PHARMACOLOGY

RECENT ADVANCES IN DERMATO-PHARMACOLOGY

Edited by

Phillip Frost, M.D.
Edward C. Gomez, M.D., Ph.D.
Nardo Zaias, M.D.

all of the

Mount Sinai Medical Center of Greater Miami
Miami Beach, Florida

S P Books Division of
SPECTRUM PUBLICATIONS, INC.
New York

RL801
R4

SPECTRUM PUBLICATIONS, INC.
175-20 Wexford Terrace, Jamaica, N.Y. 11432

Library of Congress Cataloging in Publication Data

Main entry under title:

Recent advances in dermatopharmacology.

  Includes index.
  1. Skin–Diseases–Chemotherapy. 2. Dermatopharma-
cology. I. Frost, Phillip. II. Gomez, Edward C.
III. Zaias, Nardo.
RL801.R4   615'.778   77-24605
ISBN 0-89335-022-2

Contributors

MATTHEW A. AUGUSTINE, Ph.D.
Senior Research Investigator
Squibb Institute for Research
Princeton, New Jersey

HOWARD P. BADEN, M.D.
Associate Professor of Dermatology
Harvard Medical School
Massachusetts General Hospital
Boston, Mass.

WALTER E. BARRETT, Ph.D.
Director, Short Term Research and
Development
Sandoz, Inc.
East Hanover, New Jersey

DAVID CRAM, M.D.
Assistant Professor of Dermatology
University of California School of
Medicine
San Francisco, California

C. CARNOT EVANS, M.D.
Group Leader, Section on
Dermatology
Food and Drug Administration
Rockville, Maryland

CHARLES L. FOX, JR., M.D.
Professor of Microbiology (Surgery)
College of Physicians and Surgeons
Columbia University
New York, N.Y.

PHILLIP FROST, M.D.
Chairman, Department of
Dermatology
Mount Sinai Medical Center of
Greater Miami
Miami Beach, Florida

EDWARD C. GOMEZ, M.D., Ph.D.
Departments of Dermatology and
Pathology
Mount Sinai Medical Center of
Greater Miami
Miami Beach, Florida

PETER HEBBORN, Ph.D.
Vice President for Research and
Development
Westwood Pharmaceuticals
Buffalo, N.Y.
and
Professor of Pharmacology
University of Buffalo School of
Medicine
Buffalo, N.Y.

E. LINN JONES, M.D.
Clinical Investigator
Eli Lilly and Company
Indianapolis, Indiana

LEWIS H. KAMINESTER, M.D.
Department of Dermatology
Mount Sinai Medical Center of
Greater Miami
Miami Beach, Florida

CONTRIBUTORS

A. A. KHAN, M.D.
Department of Dermatology
University of California
School of Medicine
San Francicso, Calif.

CHARLES H. KIRKPATRICK, M.D.
Head, Section of Clinical Allergy
and Hypersensitivity
National Institutes of Health
Bethesda, Maryland

ALBERT M. KLIGMAN, M.D., Ph.D.
Professor of Dermatology
University of Pennsylvania School
of Medicine
Philadelphia, Pa.

JAMES J. LEYDEN, M.D.
Department of Dermatology
University of Pennsylvania
School of Medicine
Philadelphia, Pa.

FABIO LONDOÑO, M.D.
Professor of Dermatology
Centro Dermatologico
Federico Lléras Acosta
Bogota, Columbia

HOWARD I. MAIBACH, M.D.
Professor of Dermatology
University of California School of
Medicine
San Francisco, Calif.

ARTHUR F. MICHEALIS, Ph.D.
Director, Pharmacy and
Analytical Research
Sandoz, Inc.
East Hanover, New Jersey

JOHN A. PARRISH, M.D.
Assistant Professor of Dermatology
Harvard Medical School
Massachusetts General Hospital
Boston, Mass.

DAVID A. STEVENS, M.D.
Chief, Division of Infectious Diseases
Santa Clara Valley Medical Center
San Jose, California
and
Assistant Professor
Stanford University School of
Medicine

RICHARD B. STOUGHTON, M.D.
Head, Division of Dermatology
Scripps Clinic and Research
Foundation
La Jolla, California

RONALD J. TRANCIK, Ph.D.
Research Specialist
Riker Laboratories
3M Company
Saint Paul, Minnesota

EUGENE J. VAN SCOTT, M.D.
Professor of Dermatology
Temple University School of
Medicine
Philadelphia, Pa.

GERALD N. WACHS, M.D.
Associate Medical Director
Schering Corporation
Kenilworth, New Jersey

RUEY J. YU, Ph.D.
Department of Dermatology
Temple University
School of Medicine
Philadelphia, Pa.

NARDO ZAIAS, M.D.
Department of Dermatology
Mount Sinai Medical Center of
Greater Miami
Miami Beach, Florida

Contents

CONTENTS

Preface

Needs for progress in therapy against human disease are usually related to degrees of mortality, disability, and discomfort. Most skin diseases involve some degree of disfigurement, constituting an additional compelling factor and in a large measure accounting for the traditional emphasis on therapy in dermatology. Progress in therapy against a large number of cutaneous afflictions today is urgently sought, for these are days of high expectations. Achievement of these expected advances, however, almost surely depend on progress in disciplinary dermatopharmacology.

The development of rational dermatopharmacology is considered to have been initiated early in this century after the efficacy of inorganic arsenical compounds on several diseases had been empirically established. This provided a background for the systematic development of organic arsenicals as drugs by Ehrlich, rewarded by his identification of the new antisyphilitic drug, arsphenamine, the 606th in his test series. Ehrlich's work and his objectives introduced what today is categoried as specific chemotherapy, a subject amply evident in this publication on recent advances in dermatopharmacology.

Topical therapy continues in prevalent use for most dermatologic diseases, because it makes sense to deliver a drug precisely to the seat of disease. Advances in topical therapy however require confrontation of special challenges. For example, a topically administered drug is required to move in a direction counter to that by which physiologic materials move to the skin naturally. The topical route, moreover, is often found to be cumbersome and inefficient, consequently compromising efficacy in many instances. On the other hand it diminishes risks of systemic toxicity, and hence, continues to be rational.

Dermatopharmacology today therefore deals with both topical and systemic therapy, each requiring sophisticated and disciplined approaches to the study of drugs and their effects. This book brings these aspects of dermatopharmacology into focus, assesses current states of knowledge, and provides a guide for the further pursuit of therapeutic progress against skin diseases.

Eugene J. Van Scott, MD
1977

Recent Advances in Dermatopharmacology

1

Delivery System for Griseofulvin

ARTHUR F. MICHAELIS

Griseofulvin has been the classic example of a drug whose levels in the blood have at least a rank order dependence on dissolution rate. The rate of solution is related to the number of drug particles and hence to the available surface area that can be exposed to the dissolution media. Microcrystalline griseofulvin, introduced after 1962, was shown to produce twice the blood level of an equivalent macrocrystalline dose. It is now possible to prepare a third and yet smaller crystalline-size griseofulvin consisting of a high-energy dispersion of the drug within a solid polyethylene glycol matrix. Evidence presented here which compares the particle size of the three forms of griseofulvin and their relative dissolution rates *in vitro*. The new ultramicrosize griseofulvin dissolves more rapidly than do the older forms. This allows a reduction of the dose to one-half the levels of currently marketed microsize griseofulvin dosage forms while maintaining equivalent blood levels in man.

The dissolution of drug substances is governed by the Noyes-Whitney equation:

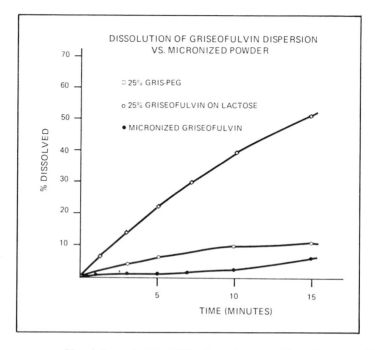

1 Dissolution of Gris-PEG dispersion vs. Microsize griseofulvin.

$$\frac{dA}{dt} = KS\,(C_s - C)$$

where dA/dt = Rate of solution
K = proportionality constant
S = Surface area
C_s = Concentration of the saturated layer at the surface of the granule or particle
C = Concentration in the bulk solution

From this equation the most readily controllable variable with regard to an oral dosage form is S, the surface area of drug that can come into contact with the dissolution solvent. Surface area is quite obviously related inversely to particle size. Hence, when griseofulvin powder was micronized in 1962, the average particle size was reduced from 10 microns to 2.7 microns. Correspondingly the surface area increased from

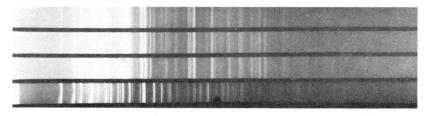

Microsize Griseofulvin mixed with milled PEG 6000

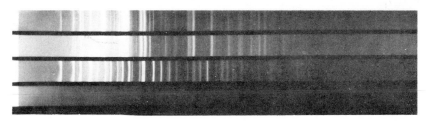

Griseofulvin-PEG 6000 Dispersion (milled)

2   X-ray diffraction patterns. (a) Microsize griseofulvin mixed with milled PEG 6000. (b) Griseofulvin-PEG 6000 dispersion (milled).

0.4 m^2/gm to 1.5 m^2/gm. This increase in surface area in turn caused an increase in dissolution rate and more efficient absorption of the drug.

It would be nice to further micronize the drug substance to produce even smaller particles, however certain other forces make that impossible. Continued grinding in a micronizer reduces particle size, but also dramatically increases the free surface energy of the particles. This energy increase causes the small particles to bind together to form aggregates which are held together so tightly that they behave as do single larger particles. Hence, there is no significant increase in dissolution rate even though individual particles may be much smaller than 2.7 μm. Additionally, the yield of particles less than approximately 1.0 μm is too low to allow for economical production operations. For this reason little has been done until recently to produce any improved dosage forms of griseofulvin.

Central to the creation of the new griseofulvin tablet is the preparation of the Griseofulvin-PEG 6000 dispersion. Chiou and Riegelman have presented several options for the preparation of such dispersions

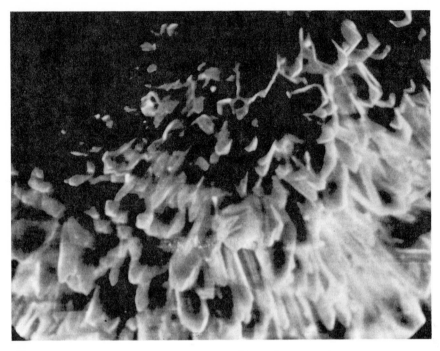

3   Macrosize griseofulvin (SEM) 1000×.

and other approaches were evaluated during the development process.[1] One particular method is used commercially to produce the dispersion. The resulting solid is an off-white waxy material, hard enough, however, to be milled, mixed, and manipulated into tablets. Dissolution characteristics of this dispersion are shown in Figure 1.

The initial concept with regard to the physical state of the griseofulvin in the dispersion was that it might have been dispersed at the molecular level. Certainly, the enhanced dissolution characteristics favored that point of view. In order to verify this theory, x-ray diffraction studies were run comparing the properly prepared dispersion to a physical mixture of microsized griseofulvin and PEG 6000 and to PEG 6000 alone. The PEG 6000 alone had no diffraction pattern, whereas the two samples containing griseofulvin exhibited line for line correspondence as shown in Figure 2. This data led to the conclusion that the state of the griseofulvin within the dispersion is not a molecular

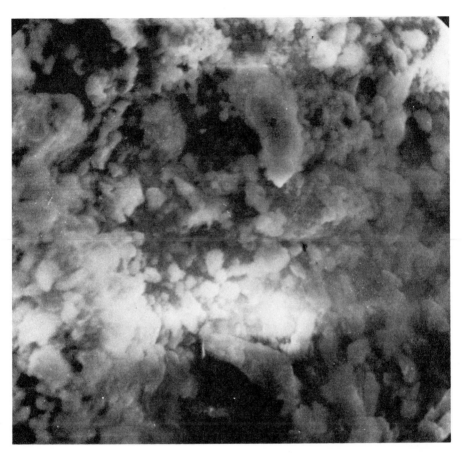

4

Microsize griseofulvin (SEM) 1000×.

scale dispersed state but rather very small crystals uniformally divided throughout the matrix.

Consideration was then given to the determination of the size of the drug particles within the matrix. Conventional methods do not allow for the determination of the size of particles within a solid matrix. Consequently, scanning electron microscopy (SEM) was used to evaluate the particle size of griseofulvin imbedded within the matrix.

In order to serve as a basis for comparison, SEMs of macrosize griseofulvin and microsize griseofulvin are shown in Figure 3 and 4

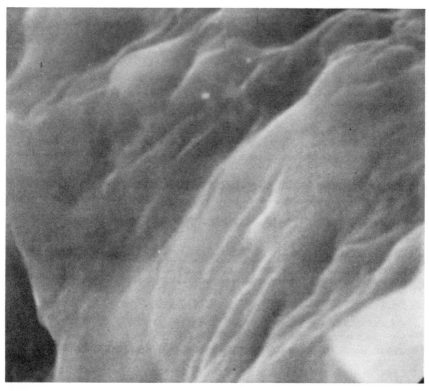

5   PEG 6000 (SEM) 10,000×.

respectively, at 1000× magnification. PEG 6000 matrix material is shown in Figure 5 at 10,000× magnification. If griseofulvin particles are mixed with molten PEG 6000 as a slurry and then solidified, the resultant material would be similar to the SEM shown in Figure 6 at 5000×. Distinct particles are visible in the surface and, of course, the dissolution properties are not satisfactory. Figure 7 depicts the surface of a piece of dispersion at 1000× and Figure 8 shows the interior (after slicing with a razor blade) at 10,000× magnification. This material shows no crystalline structure whatsoever in this internal section. Only in Figure 9 (which is the surface shown in Figure 7 but at 10,000×) do we see anything that may look like a drug particle. If we can assume the largest visible particle is a drug particle with a coating of PEG having

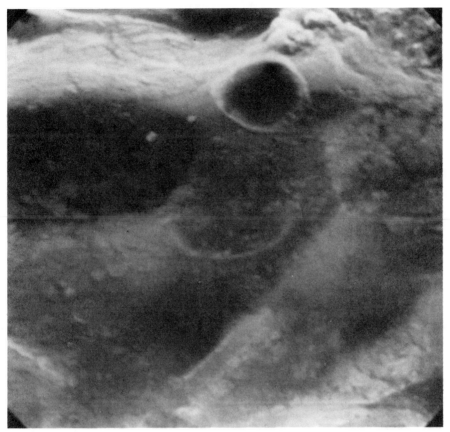

6

Microsize griseofulvin in PEG 6000 (SEM) 5000×.

no appreciable thickness, then the largest single particle seen has been 0.75 μm in its maximum dimension. Consequently, it was felt appropriate to call the new type of griseofulvin *ultramicrosize*. The estimated mean particle size for ultramicrosize particles based on a 0.75 μm maximum particle size would probably be in the order of 0.01 to 0.1 μm.

Since no griseofulvin particles were seen in the interior SEM (Figure 8) there was a need to know if any griseofulvin was there or if the drug was located at the upper surface of the dispersion as particles. An

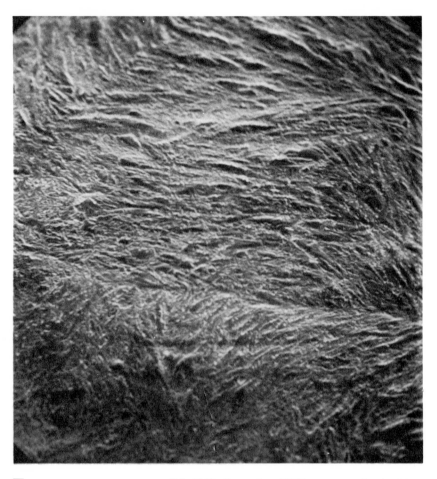

7   Gris-PEG dispersion (SEM upper surface) 1000×.

adjunct piece of apparatus to the SEM, called EDAX (energy dispersion analysis by x-ray) which allows one to pinpoint the presence of
certain atoms on the surface of an SEM sample and to a depth of a
micron or two, depending on the matrix. The handle used was the
chlorine atom which is present on the griseofulvin molecule but which
is not found in PEG 6000. Figure 10 shows a scan of the surface of the

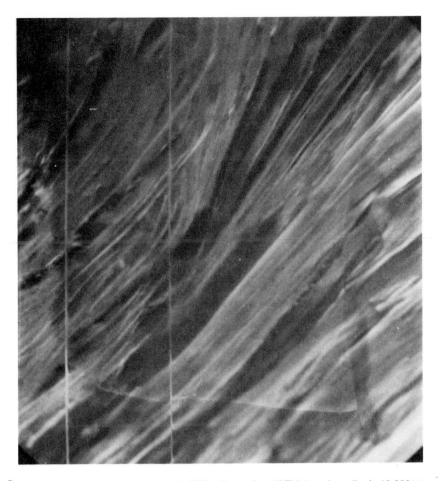

8

Gris-PEG dispersion (SEM interior slice) 10,000×.

sample and indicates a positive detection of chlorine. The sample was then scanned at the chlorine setting and showed the distribution of chlorine sites in the sample used for Figure 8. Note that although no crystals were visible at 10,000×, there is a highly uniform distribution of drug crystals throughout this typical interior sample.

The conclusion to be drawn from these studies then is that the

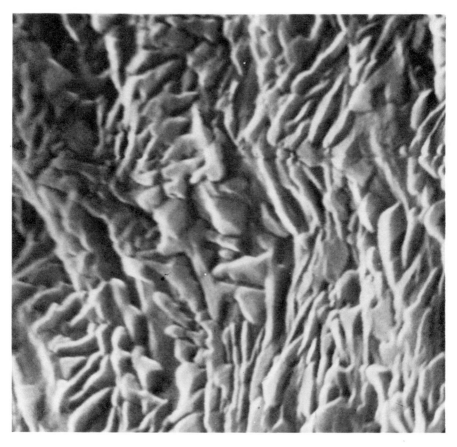

9   Gris-PEG dispersion (SEM upper surface) 10,000×.
This surface may contain particles of drug coated with PEG-6000
or it may only be a surface which cracked when the sample
was prepared.

dispersion processing of griseofulvin in PEG 6000 results in the creation of ultramicrosize particles of crystals of the drug which have a
maximum size of less than one micron. This material will dissolve
much more rapidly than will microsize griseofulvin USP and should
lead to improved absorption.

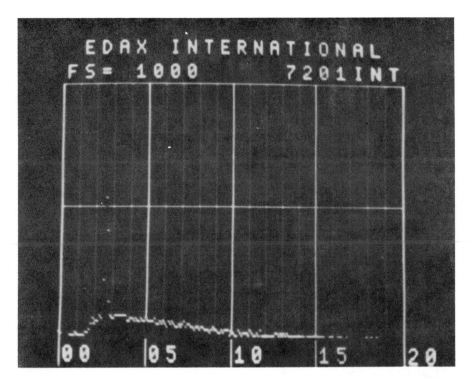

10   EDAX scan showing presence of chlorine in griseofulvin.

A suitable dosage form was needed which required that large quantities of this dispersion be prepared and that reasonably normal pharmaceutical manufacturing equipment be utilized. In order to do this a 125-mg dose tablet was formulated and the dissolution rate of griseofulvin evaluated in comparison to existing marketed products. These dissolution data are presented in Figure 12. The tablets exhibit no stability problems, can withstand temperatures of 50°C for periods of a few months, and, most importantly, show no change in dissolution rate over a period of 2 years.

In conclusion, it has been possible to prepare ultramicrosize griseofulvin crystals, within a polyethylene glycol matrix, having significantly enhanced dissolution properties. Further, tablet formula-

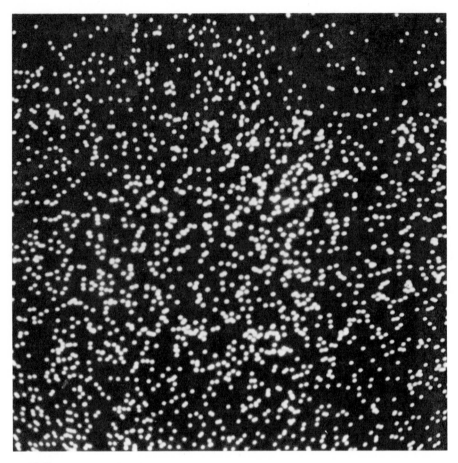

11   EDAX scan set at the chlorine detection point shows distribution of griseofulvin particles in the interior of Gris-PEG dispersion.

tion has been possible with retention of the favorable dissolution properties. The following presentation by Dr. Barrett, will show that this dissolution enhancement leads to more efficient absorption and a reduction of the recommended dose to one-half of that of the currently available microsize griseofulvin.

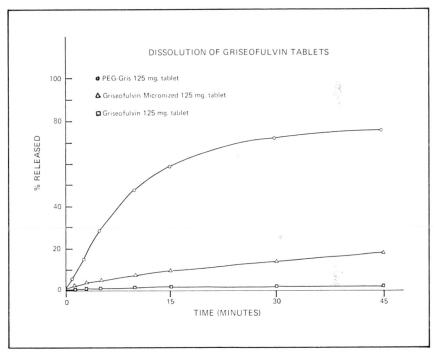

12 Dissolution of Gris-PEG tablets vs. microsize and macrosize tablets.

REFERENCES

1. W.L. Chiou and S. Riegelman. Preparation and dissolution characteristics of several fast-release dispersions of griseofulvin. *J. Pharm. Sci.* 58, 1505 (1970).

Recent Advances in Dermatopharmacology

2

The Bioavailability and Efficacy of Ultramicrosize Griseofulvin (Gris-PEG®) Tablets in Man

WALTER E. BARRETT

It is possible that in many fungus infections in man, unresponsiveness to griseofulvin therapy may be due to poor and irregular absorption of the drug (1–10).

Blood level studies carried out in several laboratories (1,4,5, 11–14) have shown that it is possible to improve intestinal absorption of griseofulvin by reducing its particle size. Blood levels equal to those resulting from a full dose of macrosize griseofulvin (10 μm plus in diameter) can be obtained with one half the dose of microsize griseofulvin (2.7 microns plus in diameter).

The reduction of particle size can be accomplished directly by several recognized techniques. The resultant fine particles may not produce the expected faster dissolution rate and better gastrointestinal absorption due to possible aggregation and agglomeration of the fine particles (11). This may be caused by the electrostatic charge that develops on the solids after milling (15).

The application of solid dispersion systems to increase rates of dissolution and oral absorption of poorly water-soluble or insoluble drugs was proposed by Sekiguchi and Obi (16) in 1961. These authors described the formation of an eutectic mixture which consisted of a physiologically inert, readily soluble carrier plus a poorly water-soluble drug. When such a solid dispersion system was exposed to water or gastrointestinal fluids, the soluble carrier was rapidly dissolved, releasing finely dispersed particles of the drug. The release of finely dispersed particles was based on the assumption that at the time of the preparation of the dispersion system, only very small particles in the submicron or micron range would be formed. Chiou and Riegelman (17) have described the *in vitro* characteristics of a solid dispersion of griseofulvin.

The *in vivo* applications of griseofulvin were demonstrated by Chiou and Riegelman in dogs and human subjects (18,19). These investigators observed that the oral administration of griseofulvin in the solid dispersion formulations gave fast and almost complete absorption, whereas only 30–60% of the commercially available microsize formulation was absorbed. In their studies they used polyethylene glycol (PEG 6000) as the dispersion carrier.

The kinetics of griseofulvin in man have been described by Rowland et al. (9).

The human bioavailability studies and the efficacy study reported in this paper were designed to corroborate and amplify the results presented by Chiou and Riegelman and to compare quantitatively the oral absorption characteristics of commercially available microsize griseofulvin tablets and ultramicrosize griseofulvin (Gris–PEG®) tablets (griseofulvin in a PEG-6000 formulation).

This comparison was made by utilizing a single-dose parallel-group bioavailability study, a single-dose crossover study, and a multiple-dose steady-state crossover study. The efficacy study was a double-blind parallel-group design.

METHODS

Parallel Group Design (Study 1).

In the first bioavaliability study, 36 male volunteers who were not confined to an institution were randomly assigned to one of three groups of equal size by means of a table of random numbers.

Group A (12 subjects) received a single oral dose of 500 mg of a commercially available formulation (tablet) of microsize griseofulvin.*

---

*Microsize griseofulvin tablets were purchased from available commercial supplies.

Group B (12 subjects) received two 125 mg ultramicrosize griseo-fulvin tablets (griseofulvin in a PEG-6000 formulation).†

Group C (12 subjects) received four 125 mg ultramicrosize griseo-fulvin tablets. All subjects received the study medications at 8:00 A.M. with 4–6 ounces of water. Blood samples for the determination of the concentration of griseofulvin in plasma were obtained at zero time and at 0.5, 1, 2, 4, 6, 8, 10, 12, and 24 hours after the oral administration of the study medications.

Single Dose Crossover Study (Study 1A)

Twelve normal healthy adult male volunteers who were not confined to an institution were selected to participate in this double-blind single-dose crossover study. Eleven subjects actually took part in this study. One subject never returned after the initial physical examination although he had been assigned a subject number. Subjects were randomly assigned to a treatment group by means of a table of random numbers.

Group I received a single oral dose of 500 mg of a commercially available microsize formulation (tablet) with 4–6 ounces of water on study day 1.

Group II received a single oral dose of 250 mg of ultramicrosize griseofulvin with 4–6 ounces of water at 8:00 A.M. on study day 1.

On study day 9, following a washout period, which extended from study day 3 to study day 8, the subjects were crossed over and received the second study medication.

Blood samples for the determination of the concentration of griseo-fulvin in the plasma were obtained at zero time and at 0.5, 1, 2, 4, 6, 8, 10, 12, 24, 36, 48, and 72 hours after the oral administration of the study medications.

Multiple Dose Steady-State Study

Eighteen normal healthy adult male volunteers who were not con-fined to an institution were selected to participate in this double-blind, multiple-dose, steady-state crossover study.

Phase I (Group A) Study Days 1 to 13. Nine subjects received an oral dose of 500 mg of a commercially available microsize griseofulvin tablet plus one matching placebo tablet at 7:00 AM and 7:00 PM with 4–6 ounces of water. The subjects received the study medica-tions on an outpatient basis except for study days 9, 11, and 13 of

†Ultramicrosize griseofulvin tablets were supplied by Sandoz, Inc.

phase I and study days 34, 36, and 38 of phase II when the study medication was given to the subjects while they were confined to the Clinical Unit of the Harris Laboratories, Inc. One subject dropped out of the study after the first study day because he could not comply with the dosage schedule. Each day the subjects reported to the investigator's office at 7:00 AM and 7:00 PM and took the study medication in the presence of the investigator or a member of his staff.

Phase I (Group B) Study Days 1 to 13. Nine subjects received two 125 mg ultramicrosize griseofulvin PEG tablets (Gris-PEG®) at 7:00 AM and 7:00 PM with 4–6 ounces of water. These subjects received the study medication on an outpatient basis, except for study days 9, 11, and 13 of phase I and study days 34, 36, and 38 of phase II when the study medication was given to the subjects while they were confined to the Clinical Unit of the Harris Laboratories, Inc. Each day the subjects reported to the investigator's office at 7:00 AM and at 7:00 PM and took the study medication in the presence of the investigator or a member of his staff.

Phase II—Study Days 26 to 38. At the end of a 12-day washout period, the two groups were crossed over and received the second study medication on study days 26 to 38 of phase II. The exact procedure followed in phase I was adhered to during phase II.

Blood samples for the determination of the concentration of griseofulvin in the plasma were obtained at zero time and at 2, 4, 6, 9, and 12 hours after the oral administration of the study medications on study days 9, 11, and 13 of phase I and study days 34, 36, and 38 of phase II. Urine samples were collected at zero time and at 0–4, 4–8, and 8–12 hours after the administration of the study medications on study days 9, 11, and 13 of phase I and on study days 34, 36, and 38 of phase II.

Efficacy Study

An efficacy study was conducted on a group of 120 soldiers who were receiving advanced army training. All of the subjects had a tinea pedis infection and had a positive KOH preparation but were free of any other significant clinical illness. Scrapings from the lesions were obtained for culture during the control period and again at the end of 4 weeks of therapy.

In this double-blind study with a parallel group design, Group A, 30 male subjects, received two 125 mg tablets of ultramicrosize griseofulvin (Gris–PEG®) b.i.d. for 4 consecutive weeks—a total daily dose of 500 mg. Group B, which consisted of 30 male subjects, received one 500 mg tablet of microsize griseofulvin plus one matching placebo tablet b.i.d. for 4 consecutive weeks—a total daily dose of 1000 mg. Group C, which consisted of 60 male subjects, received two placebo tablets b.i.d. for four consecutive weeks.

In this efficacy study, the anti-fungal activity of griseofulvin and placebo medication were evaluated in terms of the decrease in the signs of inflammation and/or infection. Safety was evaluated by: (a) clinical interpretation of the changes in vital signs and body weight; (b) the results of periodic physical examinations; and (c) type and incidence of adverse reactions encountered during therapy.

During study weeks 4 to 6, the subjects did not receive any drug but were evaluated by the investigator at the end of the sixth week.

The following parameters were evaluated at the end of study weeks 2, 4, and 6: scaling, erythema, vesiculation, overall clinical status which was made every 2 weeks and overall results of therapy. This last evaluation was made at the end of the study.

General Criteria for Inclusion in Studies

The following variables were controlled in all of the studies. All subjects were informed about the purpose and design of the studies. All gave written consent to participate in these studies. Subjects selected indicated a willingness and the motivation to cooperate in the conduct of the studies. All subjects were between the ages of 21 and 50 years, weighed between 140 and 200 pounds and were within $\pm$ 15% of the normal body weight for their frame and stature (20, 20a). In the efficacy study, the minimum age was 18 years.

Additional criteria for the inclusion of the subjects who participated in the bioavailability studies included a normal routine physical examination, complete blood count, urinalysis, and automated serum chemistries. The subjects in the efficacy study were not subjected to a battery of clinical chemistry tests because facilities for the conduct of these tests were not available at the advanced field base.

Further, all subjects were free of any significant clinical illness in the 2 weeks preceding the study; they had no surgical or medical condition which might interfere with the absorption, metabolism, or excretion of the study medications and were not taking any other medication.

In the bioavailability studies during the pretreatment phase (control period) the following parameters were studied in each subject: a 12-lead ECG, a battery of hematology tests, including a determination of the hemoglobin, hematocrit, and WBC count. Blood chemistries included a determination of the concentration of the following parameters: calcium, inorganic phosphorus, fasting blood sugar, BUN, serum uric acid, total protein, albumin, cholesterol, total bilirubin, alkaline phosphatase, LDH, and SGOT.

Subjects with abnormal values or findings were not included in these studies. These parameters were evaluated again on study day 2 in study 1. They were also evaluated again in the crossover study (study 1A) on study day 2, at the end of the washout period which was study day 8, and again on study day 10. In the multiple-dose steady-state study, these parameters were measured during the pretreatment period and on study day 13, which was the end of phase I. They were also measured on study day 25, which was the end of the washout period and again on study day 38, which was the end of phase II.

No concurrent medication was permitted during the course of these studies. For study 1 and study 1A, each subject entered the Clinical Unit of the Baltimore City Hospital the night before the study was initiated and subjects fasted overnight but were allowed water *ad lib.* No food or liquids were allowed until 4 hours after the ingestion of the study medications.

Subjects who participated in the multiple-dose steady-state study entered the Clinical Unit of the Harris Laboratories the night before study days 9, 11, and 13 of phase I and study days 34, 36, and 38 of phase II. These subjects fasted overnight but were allowed water *ad lib.* No food or liquids were allowed until 4 hours after the ingestion of the study medications on those study days when plasma and urine samples were collected, namely, study days 9, 11, and 13 of phase I and study days 34, 36, and 38 of phase II.

Analytical Methods

The plasma and urine samples were transferred using aseptic techniques to sterile plastic disposable tubes labeled with a five-digit number, frozen, and kept frozen until the time of the assay. The method employed to assay the plasma samples was a modification of the gas chromatographic method reported by Shah, Riegelman and Epstein (21) for the analysis of griseofulvin in skin, plasma, and sweat samples. Schwarz et al. (22) have recently reported upon the modification of this method. The gas chromatographic method especially with the electron capture detector was considered to be specific for griseofulvin.

The concentration of the griseofulvin metabolite, 6-demethylgriseofulvin, in the urine samples was only measured in the multiple-dose steady-state study. It was determined by the use of a liquid–solid chromatographic method described by Papp, Magyar and Schwarz (27). The work of Barnes and Boothroyd (23) indicated that the 24-hour urine sample of a patient who received one gram of griseofulvin per day contained less than 1% griseofulvin. These authors isolated and identified 6-demethylgriseofulvin as a major urinary metabolite in man. Kabasakalian et al. (12) found that in man after the administration of single doses of griseofulvin (5–500 mg), the amount of 6-demethyl-griseofulvin in human urine was proportional to the administered dose. Later, Chiou and Riegelman (19) reported that the cumulative amount excreted was a direct measure of the amount absorbed.

In the present studies, those persons who performed the chemical assays were not aware of the study medications received by any subject.

In Study 1, the statistical procedures used were the analysis of variance, the t -test against zero time and the Krushall–Wallis rank sum test.

For Study 1A, the data from the plasma samples were statistically analyzed using the analysis of variance for a crossover design. Vital signs and clinical laboratory data were analyzed by comparing the change from baseline for the two treatments. With the multiple-dose steady-state study, a repeated measurement two-period crossover design developed by Wallenstein (24) was employed to analyze the griseo-fulvin plasma concentration data. The parameters, area under the plasma level curve (trapezoidal rule), peak plasma level, and time to reach peak plasma level were also analyzed after logarithmic transformation. The crossover design was employed to analyze the changes from baseline with respect to vital signs and the clinical laboratory data.

The statistical methods used to analyze the data from the efficacy study were analysis of variance for repeated measurements design, the nonparameter analysis of variance for the repeated measurements model, and the chi square analysis for contingency tables.

RESULTS

After the concentration of griseofulvin in the plasma for each bioavailability study and the concentration of a 6-demethylgriseofulvin in urine for the multiple-dose study had been determined for each subject the following parameters were calculated for each subject and subjected to a statistical analysis: peak concentration, time to reach peak concentration, area under the plasma level curves, and urinary excretion of 6-demethylgriseofulvin for the multiple-dose study.

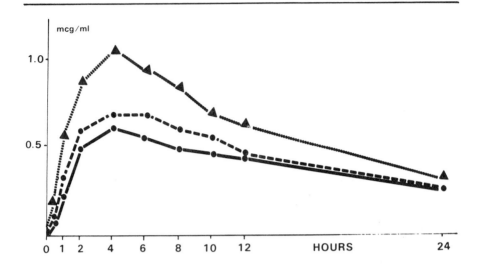

1 Study 1, the plasma concentration of griseofulvin (mcg/ml) after a single oral dose in human volunteers; gas chromatography assay. ●————● = microsize griseofulvin 500 mg; ●-——-——● = ultramicrosize griseofulvin 250 mg; and ▲--------▲ = ultramicrosize griseofulvin 500 mg.

In Study 1, a single oral dose of 250 mg of ultramicrosize griseo-fulvin produced essentially the same peak plasma concentration, the same time to reach peak concentration, and the same area under the plasma level curve as was achieved with a single oral dose of 500 mg of the microsize formulation of griseofulvin (Fig. 1). There was no statistically significant difference between the plasma levels achieved with these two study medications (Barrett et al.) (25).

Following the oral administration of a single 500 mg dose of ultra-microsize griseofulvin (Gris–PEG®) in man, the peak plasma level and the area under the plasma level curve were significantly enhanced when compared to the results obtained with a 500 mg dose of a com-mercially available microsize formulation of griseofulvin (Fig. 1). The gas chromatographic method was employed to assay the plasma samples.

In the single-dose crossover study [Study 1A, Barrett et al. (25)] an oral dose of 250 mg of ultramicrosize griseofulvin produced essentially

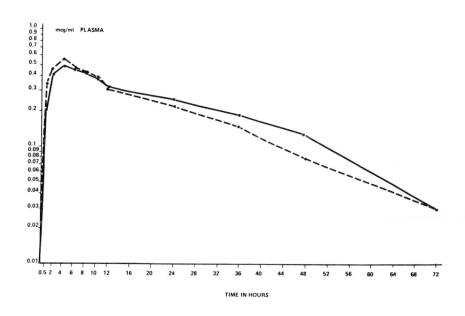

2

Study 1A, the plasma concentration of griseofulvin (mcg/ml) after a single oral dose in human volunteers; gas chromatographic assay. Log concentration vs. time in hours. O — — — — — — O = ultramicrosize griseofulvin 250 mg and ★————————★ = microsize griseofulvin 500 mg.

the same peak concentration, the same time to reach peak concentration, and the same area under the plasma level curve as was achieved with a single oral dose of 500 mg of a commercially available microsize formulation of griseofulvin. The differences between the two study medications were not significant (Fig. 2).

The numerical values for the bioavailability parameters studied in Studies 1 and 1A have been summarized in Table 1.

In Studies no. 1 and no. 1A, no adverse effects attributable to the study medications were observed on the following parameters: vital signs, ECG, hematology parameters, blood chemistry parameters, or the urinalysis tests. No adverse reactions were reported during the course of these two studies.

Table I. Bioavailability Parameters — Average Values

Study	Group[a]	N	Oral dose-(mg)	Time to peak (hr)	Peak plasma level (mcg/ml)	Area under plasma level curve (hrs mcg/m)
1	A	12	500	4.00	0.65	9.89
	B	12	250	4.67	0.80	11.18
	C	12	500	4.17	1.15	15.11
1A	I	11	500	6.10	0.51	14.36
	II	11	250	3.70	0.60	12.88

[a]A = microsize Griseofulvin (500 mg); B = ultramicrosize Griseofulvin (250 mg); C = Ultramicrosize Griseofulvin (500 mg); I = microsize Griseofulvin (500 mg); and II = ultramicrosize Griseofulvin (250 mg).

A comparison of Studies no. 1 and no. 1A indicated that in both studies there were no significant differences between treatment groups in terms of age, body weight, and height as indicated in Tables 2 and 3.

In the multiple-dose steady-state crossover study [Barrett et al. (26)]. the differences between ultramicrosize griseofulvin PEG tablets (Gris–PEG®) administered at a dose of 250 mg b.i.d. and a commercially available microsize griseofulvin formulation administered at a dose of 500 mg b.i.d. were not significant for time to reach peak concentration, peak plasma level, or area under the plasma level curve (Figs. 3 and 4).

An analysis of the data after logarithmic transformation indicated that there were no significant differences between ultramicrosize griseofulvin PEG tablets (Gris-PEG®) and the commercially available microsize griseofulvin tablets with respect to area under the plasma level curves, peak concentration, and time to reach peak concentration.

The average cumulative excretion of 6-demethylgriseofulvin over a 12-hour period on study days 9, 11, and 13 was 161.6 mg for the microsize formulation or 32% of the 500 mg oral dose administered at 7:00 AM each day. With the ultramicrosize griseofulvin PEG tablets (Gris–PEG®), the urinary excretion of 6-demethylgriseofulvin was 137.5 mg or 55% of the 250 mg oral dose administered at 7:00 AM each day (Figs. 5 and 6).

There was no statistically significant difference between treatment groups with respect to age, body weight, or height at the pretreatment control period (Table 4).

Table II. Study no. 1 — Summary of Background Data
Mean ± Standard Deviation

Drug group[a]	Age (years)	Weight [lbs (kg)]	Height In [inches (cm)]
A	24.1 ± 2.4	160.3 ± 15.8 (72.71 ± 7.1 kg)	69.4 ± 2.4 (176.2 ± 6.1 cm)
B	27.2 ± 5.3	160.4 ± 16.4 (72.76 ± 7.4 kg)	69.1 ± 3.5 (175.5 ± 8.8 cm)
C	24.1 ± 2.0	156.5 ± 15.9 (70.99 ± 7.2 kg)	70.4 ± 2.0 (178.8 ± 5.1 cm)

[a]A = microsize griseofulvin (500 mg); B = ultramicrosize griseofulvin (250 mg); and C = ultramicrosize griseofulvin (500 mg).

Table III. Study no 1A — Summary of Background Data
Mean ± Standard Deviation

Drug group[a]	N	Age (years)	Weight [lbs (kg)]	Height In [inches (cm)]
I	5	25.6 ± 3.5	152.0 ± 9.2 (68.95 ± 4.2 kg)	70.2 ± 1.9 (178.3 ± 4.8 cm)
II	6	22.3 ± 1.0	157.6 ± 5.1 (71.49 ± 2.3 kg)	70.7 ± 2.7 (179.5 ± 6.8 cm)

[a]I = microsize griseofulvin (500 mg) and II = ultramicrosize griseofulvin (250 mg).

Neither study medication had an adverse effect on the vital signs, ECG, blood chemistries, or urinalysis tests.

The efficacy study conducted in soldiers who had a tinea pedis infection was conducted in such a manner that it did not interfere with the participation of the subjects in the advanced army training program at the field camp. A culture of the scrapings obtained from the lesions indicated a positive culture in 64% of the subjects. The infecting organisms were found to be E. floccosum or T. mentagrophytes or both. No attempts were made to institute a local hygienic treatment of the tinea

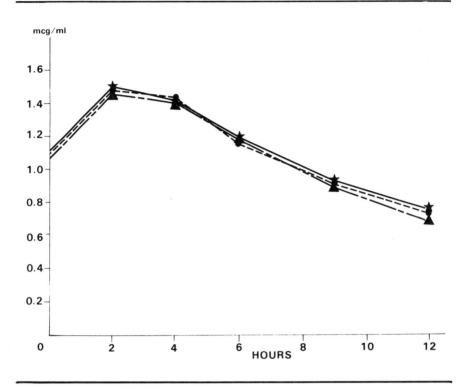

3 The average plasma concentration of griseofulvin (mcg/ml) produced by microsized griseofulvin tablets (500 mg b.i.d.) following the administration of multiple oral doses to human volunteers (study days 9, 11, and 13). ★————————★ = day 9; ● — — — — — ● = day 11; and ▲ — — · — — ▲ = day 13.

pedis infection. In spite of the adverse field conditions which existed at this army field camp, both the ultramicrosize griseofulvin treated group (Gris–PEG®) and the group treated with the commercially available microsize griseofulvin exhibited a significantly greater improvement than did the placebo treated group. A summary of the results obtained is presented in Table 5. A total of 95 patients were included in the analysis of the efficacy data.

The patients in each treatment group took essentially the same number of tablets; the group treated with microsize griseofulvin took

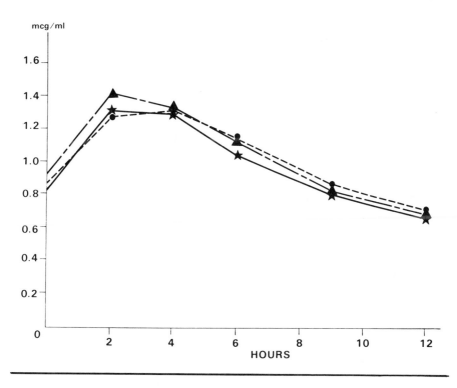

4

The average plasma concentration of griseofulvin (mcg/ml) produced by ultramicrosize griseofulvin tablets (Gris-PEG®, 250 mg b.i.d.) following the administration of multiple oral doses to human volunteers (study days 9, 11, and 13).
★————————★ = day 9; ●———————● = day 11; and ▲——— - ———▲ = day 13.

an average of 57.10 tablets per 2-week period; the placebo group 57.02 tablets per 2-week period; and the group treated with ultramicrosize griseofulvin (Gris–PEG®) 56.86 tablets per 2-week period. Each subject received a 2-week supply of medication plus two additional packets for one additional day of treatment for use in the event they were unable to see the investigator at the end of the 2-week period. Each dose of the drug was sealed in an individual packet. At the end of each 2-week period the patients received a new 2-week supply of the drug. The com-

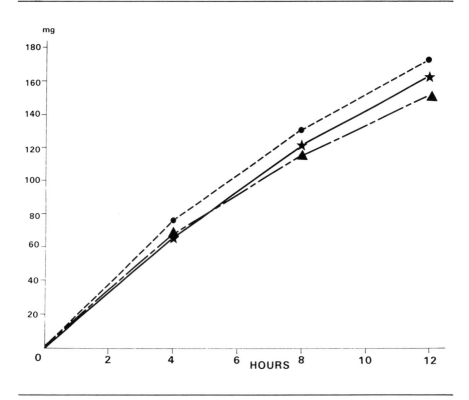

5 Average urinary excretion of 6-demethylgriseofulvin for study days 9, 11, and 13 following the administration of multiple oral doses of microsize griseofulvin tablets (500 mg b.i.d.) to human volunteers ★————————★ = day 9; ● ------- ● = day 11; and ▲————·————▲ = day 13.

pliance of the patients in adhering to the prescribed dosage schedule was excellent.

There was no significant difference observed between ultramicrosize griseofulvin (250 mg b.i.d.) and microsize griseofulvin (500 mg b.i.d.) in terms of clinical efficacy as measured by several efficacy parameters. No complete cures were obtained with the commercially available microsize griseofulvin or the ultramicrosize griseofulvin (Gris–PEG®) when

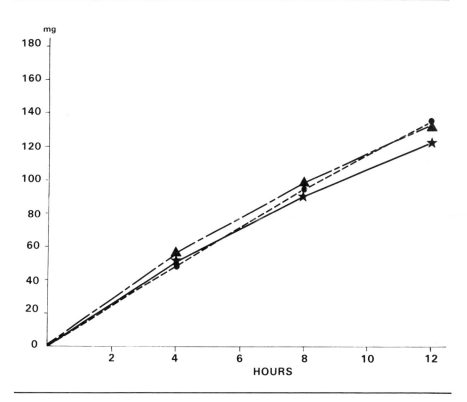

6 Average urinary excretion of 6-demethylgriseofulvin for study days 9, 11, and 13 following the administration of multiple oral doses of ultra microsize griseofulvin tablets (Gris-PEG®, 250 mg b.i.d.) to human volunteers. ★————————★ = day 9; ● - - - - - - - - ● = day 11; and ▲————·——▲ = day 13.

administered for 4 consecutive weeks under the adverse field conditions which were present at the advanced army training field base.

CONCLUSIONS

The single dose studies demonstrated that an oral dose of 250 mg of ultramicrosize griseofulvin (Gris–PEG®) tablets was biologically

Table IV. Multiple-Dose Steady-State Crossover Study;
Background Data For The Control Period
Average Value ± Standard Deviation

Parameter	Treatment	
	Group A[a]	Group B[b]
Age (years)	M = 23.89 ± 2.98	M = 24.11 ± 2.76
Body weight		
lbs.	M = 169.2 ± 12.62	M = 162.0 ± 12.31
kg	M = 76.75 ± 5.72	M = 73.48 ± 5.58
Height		
inches	M = 71.78 ± 2.95	M = 71.00 ± 2.40
cm	M = 182.32 ± 7.49	M = 180.34 ± 6.10

[a]Subjects were given ultramicrosize griseofulvin (Gris-PEG®) in phase I of the study and microsize griseofulvin in phase II.
[b]Subjects were given microsize griseofulvin in phase I of the study and ultramicrosize griseofulvin (Gris-PEG®) in phase II.

equivalent to an oral dose of 500 mg of microsize griseofulvin tablets.

Data obtained from the multiple-dose steady-state crossover study indicated that the bioavailability of 250 mg b.i.d. of ultramicrosize griseofulvin (Gris–PEG®) tablets at the steady state of dosing was equivalent to the bioavailability of 500 mg b.i.d. of microsize griseofulvin tablets at the steady state of dosing.

A double-blind clinical efficacy study demonstrated a statistically significant clinical improvement of a tinea pedis infection in patients who received ultramicrosize griseofulvin (Gris–PEG®) tablets, 250 mg b.i.d., or microsize griseofulvin tablets,   500 mg b.i.d., compared to patients who received placebo tablets b.i.d.

There was no significant difference in clinical efficacy, as judged by several parameters, between ultramicrosize griseofulvin (Gris–PEG®) tablets, 250 mg b.i.d., and microsize griseofulvin tablets, 500 mg. b.i.d.

The results from all of the studies indicated that the PEG 6000 formulation significantly enhanced the oral absorption of griseofulvin in man.

Table V. Summary of Efficacy Data Analysis

Parameter	N	Pre	Week 2	Week 4	
1. Scaling[a]					
Grisactin	20	1.75	-0.05	-0.40^d	⎤ e
Placebo	49	2.10	-0.06	0.12	⎦
Gris-PEG®	26	2.15	-0.27	-0.62^f	⎤ e
2. Erythema[a]					
Grisactin	20	1.55	-0.30^f	-0.85^f	
Placebo	49	1.71	-0.57	-0.57^f	
Gris-PEG®	26	0.69	-0.69^f	-1.08^f	
3. Vesiculation[a]					
Grisactin	20	0.10	0.00	0.00	
Placebo	49	0.20	0.16	0.24^f	
Gris-PEG®	26	0.27	0.00	0.00	
4. Overall clinical status[b]					
Grisactin	20	–	0.70	1.35	⎤ e
Placebo	49	–	0.67	0.71	⎦
Gris-PEG®	26	–	1.35 ⎤ e	1.73	⎤ e
5. Overall results of therapy[c]					
Grisactin	20			3.00	⎤ e
Placebo	48			2.25	⎦
Gris-PEG®	26			3.27	⎤ e

[a]The following grading scheme was employed for parameters 1, 2, and 3:0 = Absent; 1 = Slight; 2 = Moderate; 3 = Marked; and 4 = Severe.
[b]The following grading scheme was employed for parameter 4: 0 = None; 1 = Slight; 2 = Moderate; and 3 = Marked clinical improvement.
[c]The following grading scheme was employed for parameter 5: 1 = Worse; 2 = Unchanged; 3 = Poor; 4 = Fair; 5 = Good; and 6 = Excellent.
[d]$p = 0.05$ - significant change from control value.
⎤ [e] = signficant difference between treatment groups.
[f]$p = 0.01$ - significant change from control value.

ACKNOWLEDGMENTS

The single dose bioavailability studies were conducted under the medical supervision of Dr. Joseph Bianchine* at the Clinical Pharmacology unit of the Baltimore City Hospital, Baltimore, Maryland.

The multiple dose steady state crossover study was conducted under the medical supervision of Dr. John J. Hanigan, Harris Laboratories, Inc., Lincoln, Nebraska.

The efficacy study was conducted by Dr. William H. Eaglstein and Professor David Taplin, Department of Dermatology, University of Miami, School of Medicine, Miami, Florida.

The assay of the plasma and urine samples was conducted under the supervision of Hans Schwarz, Ph.D., Director of Drug Metabolism Unit, Biological Research, Pharmaceutical Research & Development, Sandoz, Inc., East Hanover, New Jersey. The modification of the existing methods to allow one to assay a large number of samples was also carried out under the direction of Dr. Hans Schwarz.

The statistical analysis of the data generated by these studies was performed by Hans Mueller, Ph.D., and Sylvan Wallenstein, Ph.D.,** of the Department of Research Data Services, Pharmaceutical Research and Development, Sandoz, Inc., East Hanover, New Jersey.

REFERENCES

1. R.M. Atkinson, C. Bedford, K.J. Child, and E.G. Tomich. Effect of particle size on blood griseofulvin levels in man. *Nature* 193, 588–589 (1962).
2. R.G. Crounse. Human pharmacology of griseofulvin: The effect of fat intake on gastrointestinal absorption. *J. Invest. Derm.* 37, 529–533 (1961).
3. W.A.M. Duncan, G. MacDonald, and M.J. Thornton. Some factors influencing the absorption of griseofulvin from the gastrointestinal tract. *J. Pharm. Pharmacol.* 14, 217–224 (1962).
4. A. Gonzales-Ochoa, and M. Ahumada-Padilla. New schemes in the treatment of dermatophytoses with griseofulvin. *Arch. Derm.* (*Chicago*) 81, 833–837 (1960).

---

*Present Address: Professor and Chairman of The Department of Pharmacology, Ohio State University, School of Medicine, 333 West 10th Avenue, Columbus, Ohio 43210.

**Present address: Columbia University, School of Public Health, Department of Statistics, 600 W. 68th Street, N.Y., N.Y. 10032.

5. M. Kraml, J. Dubuc, and D. Beall. Gastrointestinal absorption of griseofulvin. I. Effects of particle size, addition of surfactants, and corn oil on the level of griseofulvin in the serum of rats. *Canad. J. Biochem. Physiol.* 40. 1449–1451 (1962).
6. M. Kraml, J. Dubuc, and R. Gaudry. Gastrointestinal absorption of griseofulvin. II. Influence of particle size in man. *Antibiot. Chemother.* (N.Y.) 12, 239–242 (1962).
7. E.G. McNall. Metabolic studies on griseofulvin and its mechanism of action. *Antibiot. Ann.* 7, 674–679. 1957–1960.
8. S. Riegelman, W.L. Epstein, and R.J. Dayan. "Absorption. Metabolism and Elimination of Griseofulvin in Man." Presented at the American Pharmaceutical Association Convention, 1962, Las Vegas, Nevada.
9. M. Rowland, S. Riegelman, and W.L. Epstein. Absorption kinetics of griseofulvin in man. *J. Pharm. Sci.* 57, 984–989 (1968).
10. G.D. Weinstein, and H. Blank. Quantitative determination of griseofulvin by a spectrophotofluorometric assay. *Arch. Derm.* (*Chicago*) 81, 746–749 (1960).
11. R.M. Atkinson, C. Bedford, K.J. Child, and E.G. Tomich. The effect of griseofulvin particle size on blood levels in man. *Antibiot. Chemother.* (N.Y.) 12, 232–238 (1962).
12. P. Kabasakalian, M. Kats, B. Rosenkrantz, and E. Townley. Parameters affecting absorption of griseofulvin in a human subject using urinary metabolite excretion data. *J. Pharm. Sci.* 59, 595–600 (1970).
13. M. Kraml, J. Dubuc, and D. Dvornik. Gastrointestinal absorption of griseofulvin. *Arch. Dermatol.* 87, 179–182 (1963).
14. J.R. Marvel, D.A. Schlichting, C. Denton, E.J. Levy, and, M.M. Cahn. The effect of surfactant and of particle size on griseofulvin plasma levels. *J. Invest. Dermatol.* 42, 197–203 (1964).
15. S. Lin, J. Menig, and L. Lachman. Interdependence of physiological surfactant and drug particle size on the dissolution behavior of water-insoluble drugs. *J. Pharm. Sci.* 57, 2143–2148 (1968).
16. K. Sekiguchi, and N. Obi. Studies of absorption of eutectic mixture. I. A comparison of the behavior of eutectic mixture of sulfathiazole and that of ordinary sulfathiazole in man. *Chem. Pharm. Bull.* 9, 866–872 (1961).
17. W.L. Chiou, and S. Riegelman. Preparation and dissolution characteristics of several fast-release solid dispersions of griseofulvin. *J. Pharm. Sci.* 58, 1505–1510 (1969).
18. W.L. Chiou, and S. Riegelman. Oral absorption of griseofulvin in dogs: Increased absorption via solid dispersion of polyethylene Glycol 6000. *J. Pharm. Sci.* 59, 937–942 (1970).
19. W.L. Chiou, and S. Riegelman. Absorption characteristics of solid dispersed and micronized griseofulvin in man. *J. Pharm. Sci.* 60. 1376–1380 (1971).
20. Metropolitan Life Insurance Company, Metropolitan Life Insurance

Company Tables Modified by Sandoz to Reflect Mid-Point of Weight Range by Height and Frame. *Statistical Bulletin* 40, 1–4 (1959).

20a. Metropolitan Life Insurance Company. Metropolitan Life Insurance Company Tables Modified by Sandoz to Reflect Mid-Point of Weight Range by Height and Frame, *Statistical Bulletin* 47, 1 (1966).

21. V.P. Shah, S. Riegelman, W.L. Epstein. Determination of griseofulvin in skin, plasma and sweat. *J. Pharm. Sci.* 61, 634–636 (1972).

22. H.J. Schwarz, B.A. Waldman, and V. Madrid. GLC determination of griseofulvin in human plasma. *J. Pharm. Sci.* 65 (No. 3), 370–372 (1976).

23. M.J. Barnes, B. Boothroyd. The metabolism of griseofulvin in mammals. *Biochem. J.* 78, 41–43 (1961).

24. S. Wallenstein. The Two-Period Repeated Measurements Change-Over Design With Application to Bioavailability Trials. Presented at Allied Social Science Association, National Convention Program, December 1973, New York.

25. W.E. Barrett, J. Bianchine. The bioavailability of ultramicrosize griseofulvin (Gris–PEG®) tablets in man. *Current Therapeutic Research* 18 (No. 3), 501–509 (1975).

26. W.E. Barrett, and John J. Hanigan. The bioavailability of griseofulvin PEG ultramicrosize (Gris–PEG®) tablets in man under steady state conditions. *Current Therapeutic Research* 18 (No. 3), 491–500 (1975).

27. E. Papp, K. Magyar, and H.J. Schwarz. Liquid-solid chromatographic determination of 6-demethylgriseofulvin in urine. *J. Pharm. Sci.* 65 (No. 3), 441–443 (1976).

Recent Advances in Dermatopharmacology

3

Topical Treatment of Superficial Mycoses with Two New Antifungal Agents: Clotrimazole (1 per cent) Lotion and Miconazole (2 per cent) Cream

NARDO ZAIAS

ANTIMYCOTIC AGENTS: PAST, PRESENT, AND FUTURE

While working with animals in 1959, Gentles broke the existing antifungal deadlock by introducing griseofulvin. This antifungal agent, although known as a therapeutic agent for plants, had not been considered for human use until many investigators followed Gentles' obvious hint. After 15 years of human use it still remains the best and safest systemically administered drug for treatment of infections caused by dermatophytic fungi, the only genera against which it is effective.

This unique antifungal specificity, which was a breakthrough when demonstrated in 1959, is, in 1976, the achilles heel of dermatophytic fungi. Through its reign, 1959–1974, griseofulvin totally dominated ringworm therapy. Although other chemicals were found which had significant antifungal activity, none could be used systemically. Various topically applied agents were active but could not be used systemically. Various topically applied agents were active but had to be discontinued because of irritative properties. In 1963 or earlier, thiabendazole enjoyed the unique characteristic of being both safe and as effective as

35

Table I. Double-Blind Studies of Clotrimazole Lotion and
Miconazole Cream in the Treatment of *Tinea Versicolor*

Preparation[a]	Number of patients treated	Number of patients cured[b]
Clotrimazole Lotion 1%	35	30 (86%)
Clotrimazole Placebo Lotion	33	17 (52%)
Miconazole Cream 2%	38	35 (92%)
Miconazole Placebo Cream	41	5 (12%)

[a]Preparation applied once each day for 14 days.
[b]Clinical and mycological cure 14 days after the cessation of treatment.

systemic griseofulvin against dermatophytes when topically applied; it was, however, never reported as topically effective until 1974. The study of the substituted imidazoles led to the realization that one drug could be effective against a variety of fungi and resulted in the formulation   of broad-spectrum, topically effective antifungal preparations.

This presentation discusses the relative efficacy of two of the leading broad-spectrum antimycotics: clotrimazole (Bayer) and miconazole (J & J).

TINEA VERSICOLOR

Although various medications have been found to be beneficial in the treatment of this most ubiquitous fungi, it is not easy to eradicate and usually requires prolonged or repeated treatment. In the past, sodium thiosulfate was proved effective, but the strong odor and the required prolonged treatment make it impractical. Selenium sulfide (1 or 2%) is another effective agent but data as to its effectiveness and follow-up treatment are scarce.

Table 1 presents data from double-blind studies on the efficacy of clotrimazole and miconazole after 14 days treatment and a similar period of post treatment follow-up. Both drugs are very efficacious: clotrimazole lotion, 86% clinically and mycologically cured as compared to 52% with the vehicle; miconazole cream 92%, cured as compared to 12% with the vehicle.

Table II. Double-Blind Studies of Clotrimazole Lotion and
Miconazole Cream in the Treatment of Cutaneous Candidiasis[a]

Preparation[a]	Number of patients treated	Number of patients cured[b]
Clotrimazole Lotion 1%	56	49 (88%)
Clotrimazole Placebo Lotion	43	14 (33%)
Miconazole Cream 2%	13	9 (70%)
Miconazole Placebo Cream	11	4 (36%)

[a]Treatment period 14 days. All yeasts identified as candida albicans by germ tube method.
[b]Clinical and mycological cure 14 days after the cessation of treatment.

Review of the literature concerning the beneficial effect of these
drugs against tinea versicolor as reported by various investigators in
open (not double-blind) studies shows results comparable to the results
obtained in the double-blind studies described above.

CUTANEOUS CANDIDIASIS

Cutaneous candidiasis is an opportunistic infection of the skin
surface in that quantities of the infecting organism are continually
shed from the GI tract and dispersed over the body surface without
causing disease. In the intertrigenous areas, the yeast grow, yet are
kept under control by the antimicrobial environment and undefined
host factors present on the skin surface. When this delicate balance is
upset, the organism thrives and clinical lesions result.

Presently, the polyene antibiotics (nystatin, trichomycin, pimaricin,
hamycin, and candidiacin) are widely used in the treatment of this
condition and are excellent therapeutic agents. It can be expected that
intertrigenous lesions should clear within 2 weeks of treatment and stay
clear thereafter. Both 1% clotrimazole lotion and 2% miconazole cream
(Table 2) are efficacious against *C. albicans* in *in vivo* double-blind
studies (1). Although the number of cases treated is as yet small, the
results are comparable to those obtained in open studies.

The slight differences in cure rates, 88% for clotrimazole lotion vs.
70% for miconazole cream, may reflect differences in efficacy due to the
different vehicles rather than the active ingredients. This should be
further studied by comparing these agents in more similar vehicles.

Table III. Double-Blind Studies of Clotrimazole Lotion and
Miconazole Cream in the Treatment of *T. cruris or corporis*[a]

Preparation	Number of patients treated	Number of patients cured[b]
Clotrimazole Lotion 1%	34	33 (97%)
Clotrimazole Placebo Lotion	39	5 (15%)
Miconazole Cream 2%	52	48 (92%)
Miconazole Placebo Cream	52	8 (15%)

[a]Treatment period was 28 days.
[b]Clinical and mycological cure 14 days after cessation of therapy.

DERMATOPHYTOSIS

In this disease one must consider the various clinical types separately, since the duration of treatment required and the fungal involvement is different in each. Thus, we must separate (1) hair involvement (*T. capitis, Tinea barbae, Majjocci's granuloma*), (2) volar skin involvement (*Tinea pedis, Tinea manum*), (3) nail involvement (onychomycosis), and (4) glaborous skin involvement (*Tinea corporis, Tinea cruris*). The record of cures in each of the categories is well known since there is 15 years of experience of treatment with systemic griseofulvin.

As yet, significant double blind studies in *Tinea capitis* and onychomycosis are unavailable.

TINEA CORPORIS—TINEA CRURIS

Both 1% clotrimazole lotion and 2% miconazole cream are highly effective agents for these conditions. Table 3 summarizes our experience with these agents. A 92% cure rate was found with miconazole. Again, these results corroborate the findings of other investigators in open studies.

TINEA PEDIS

Both clotrimazole lotion and miconazole cream are highly effective as compared to systemic griseofulvin. Table 4 summarizes results of a double-blind study with clotrimazole lotion in which the treatment

Table IV. Double-Blind Studies of Clotrimazole Lotion and
Miconazole Cream in the Treatment of *T. pedis*[a]

Preparation	Number of patients treated	Number of patients cured[b]
Clotrimazole Lotion 1%	16	12 (75%)
Clotrimazole Placebo Lotion	17	6 (35%)
Miconazole Cream 2%	50	44 (88%)
Miconazole Placebo Cream	50	5 (10%)

[a]Treatment period was 28 days.
[b]Clinical and mycological cure 14 days after cessation of treatment in clotrimazole study and
20 days after cessation of treatment in miconazole study.

time was 28 days and the patients were followed for 14 days (clotrimazole) or 20 days (miconazole). A cure rate of 75% was obtained with
clotrimazole and 88% with miconazole.

SIDE EFFECTS

The worldwide experience with both clotrimazole lotion and
miconazole cream show these antibiotics to be safe with an insig-
nificant local irritancy and no systemic effects.

DISCUSSION

Since the introduction of griseofulvin no topical agent has ap-
proached its efficacy in the treatment of dermatophyte infections.
Present data indicate that clotrimazole and miconazole not only have
about the same level of efficacy as griseofulvin against such organisms
but also have a broader spectrum, being effective against *Candida
albicans* and the causative agent of *Tinea versicolor*. These characteristics make them ideal agents for the treatment of infections of uncertain
fungal etiology or "mixed infections."

REFERENCES

1. N. Zaias and F. Battistini. Superficial mycoses—Treatment with new
   broad spectrum antifungal agent, 1% clotrimazole solution. *Archives of
   Dermatology*. (in press 1977).

Recent Advances in Dermatopharmacology

4

Pharmacodynamics of Silver Sulfadiazine and Related Topical Antimicrobial Agents

CHARLES L. FOX, JR.

After successful resuscitation, burns are susceptible to infection, especially with *Pseudomonas aeruginosa;* purulence is obvious, and the peculiar, foul odor of pseudomonas cultures permeats the wounds and the patient's room. Conversion of partial-thickness burns to full-thickness burns delays healing; bacterial invasion of the blood and vital organs causes a high incidence of fatal burn wound sepsis. Because of vascular blockage resulting from hypercoagulation and thrombosis in the microcirculation of the burned skin (1), systemic antibiotics are unable to reach the wounds. Accordingly, topical antibacterial agents such as silver nitrate, sulfamylon, betadine, gentamicin, and silver sulfadiazine have been used to suppress or eliminate bacteria in the wound and expediate healing (2–5).

World wide clinical trials (6–18) have shown that effective control of infection with few disadvantages is obtained with 1% silver sulfadiazine water-miscible cream. The wide spectrum of antibacterial action eliminates gram negative and gram positive bacteria and also fungal infections (19), which often gain access to the burn wound.

This type of control of local infection alters the manner of eschar separation. Heretofore proliferating bacteria and their enzymes played a large part in the removal of the eschar. With silver sulfadiazine, little if any bacterial growth occurs and the eschar is dissolved gradually by the proteolytic enzymes present in the thermally killed cells and exudate. The proteolytic activity enhanced by covering dressings produces a soft, disintegrating eschar which ultimately becomes a gelatinous, yellow exudate which looks purulent but is usually devoid of bacteria and leukocytes (14,15).

USE OF SILVER SULFADIAZINE CREAM

The cream is applied with a gloved hand, and should cover the burned tissues with a layer approximately 2 to 4 mm in thickness. Application to the wounds is not painful and is done with great care to get the medication into all the interstices and crevices in the burned skin. Although the anointed wounds can be left exposed as described by Baxter (6) and McDougal (11), many patients are usually more comfortable with an occlusive dressing consisting of two layers of fine mesh gauze placed over the anointed burns, then a second bulky layer of gauze pads, and finally secured with a firm Kling bandage. Such a dressing, which is comfortable and reduces evaporative water loss can remain for 24 to 48 hours without replacement.

Although the dressings are removed easily because they remain moist and do not adhere, washing in a 0.6% sodium bicarbonate solution (nonsterile at 37°C) is a comfortable and effective method of facilitating removal and assisting in the cleansing and separation of necrotic tissue. Inasmuch as only loose pieces of eschar are trimmed off, no bleeding should occur. The face and such areas as the genitalia are not bandaged but, rather, are covered frequently with the ointment.

This therapy appears to encourage maximal regeneration of epithelium and healing of the wounds from surviving epithelial islands. Often full-thickness destruction is not total, and this therapy, which is continued until the wound is closed, has resulted in the healing of many apparently deep burns without skin grafting. An illustration of this is shown in Fig. 1.

Wounds which are not healed in 4 weeks require skin grafts. When large areas of full-thickness burns are mixed with areas that are healing, the use of homografts (or heterografts) should be tried. These can cover both full-thickness and adjacent partial-thickness burns and reduce exudation without inhibiting healing. They serve as an effective and comfortable temporary dressing which requires changing at 5-day

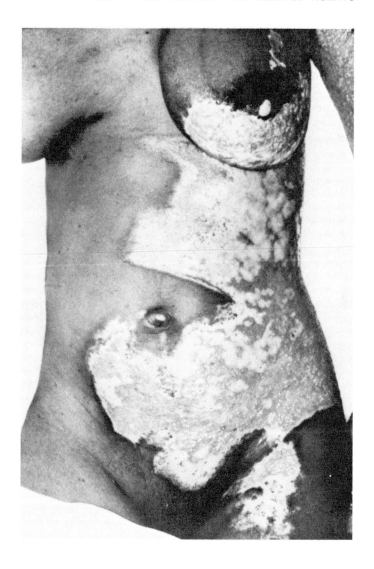

1

Islands of epithelial regeneration after 3 weeks of topical AgSD therapy.

intervals. During that time, full-thickness areas are made ready for autogenous skin grafts, and maximal reepithialization occurs.

In preparation for (and after) skin grafting, a thin layer of silver sulfadiazine ointment is spread on fine mesh gauze and this is applied over the homografts and later over autografts to prevent any infection which might reduce their take (16).

Systemic antibiotics are usually not used. If intermittent elevations of temperature, a sign of systemic infection, occur, vigorous appropriate antibiotic therapy should be instituted promptly. Moderate fever frequently occurs as the eschar disintegrates and dissolves; this is not, in itself, an indication for supplementary antibiotic therapy. Supplementary zinc therapy (30), as described below, is clearly indicated in such cases to improve wound healing.

DESCRIPTION

Silver sulfadiazine is made by substituting a silver ion for the ionizable H^+ in sulfadiazine. The resulting product is a white powder which is only very slightly soluble in water (less than 0.2 mg/100 ml) and most organic solvents. This compound does not darken on exposure to light. The minimum inhibitory concentration for pseudomonas and other organisms is extremely low, 0.5 μmoles/100 ml compared to 2.00 μmoles/100 ml for sulfadiazine. Silvadene® cream contains 1% silver sulfadiazine powder in a soft, white, water-miscible vehicle which is made with just enough drag to permit comfortable application to tender wound surfaces.

The pharmacologic reactions of silver sulfadiazine differ from sulfadiazine in several important respects:

1. Its efficacy is not blocked by *para*-aminobenzoic acid or other wound constituents or metabolites.

2. Its broad antimicrobial action inhibits many species of bacteria, herpes virus (17), fungi, such as *Candida albicans* (18), and *Treponema pallidum* (19). This wide range of infectious agents is relatively or totally resistant to sulfadiazine and the other antimicrobial agents used in topical therapy.

3. Its mode of action is distinctly different from that of sulfadiazine. The silver sulfadiazine reacts rapidly with DNA and bacteria which bind the silver and release the sulfadiazine moiety. As shown in Figure 2, the silver is bonded between the paired bases of the nucleic acids. In contrast, none of the sulfadiazine is detectable in either the DNA or the microorganisms (20).

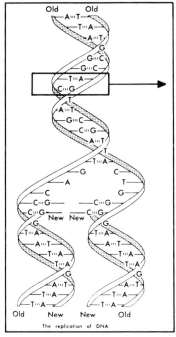

The replication of DNA.

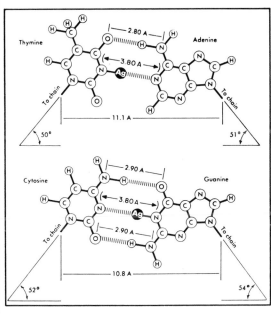

2

The binding of silver by deoxyribonucleic acid. On the left is shown the double helix of deoxyribonucleic acid. The basis T....A and C....G are joined by hydrogen bonds. In addition, as pointed out by Wilkins, there is hydrophobic bonding in aqueous media because the flat sides of the bases cannot bind water molecules. Cell replication is preceded by separation of the two strands, as indicated. On the right is an enlarged view of one section of the model showing the site where the silver is substituted for the hydrogen bond between the nitrogens of the bases, as described by Jensen and Davidson (39). Inasmuch as the N–Ag....N distance should be about 3.8 Å whereas an N–N....H distance is about 3.0 Å a certain amount of distortion of the Watson–Crick structure would occur (14).

In the test tube, soluble silver nitrate acts similarly, but in wounds the chloride and other anions in extracellular fluid combine instantly with, and thereby remove, the silver. This reaction explains the sodium and chloride depletion associated with silver nitrate therapy. In contrast, silver sulfadiazine reacts extremely slowly with chloride, does not stain, and by virtue of its low solubility forms an antimicrobial reservoir in the burned tissues. This reservoir continuously delivers low levels of silver sulfadiazine for long periods, thereby killing the bacteria present and inhibiting their proliferation without, however, preventing regeneration of surviving epithelial cells. It might be wondered how it is possible for the silver sulfadiazine, which bonds to DNA, to avoid bonding with the DNA in epithelial cells. The answer is provided by the analyses of Watson (21) who showed that epithelial cells contain approximately 800 times more DNA per cell than microbial cells. Thus, in view of the low solubility of the silver sulfadiazine it is not possible to achieve any significant bonding of the DNA of the epithelial cells which thereby continue to proliferate.

Inasmuch as less than 10% of the sulfadiazine from the silver sulfadiazine in the wound is released and absorbed, only low levels of sulfadiazine occur in blood and urine. Analyses of extensively burned patients have shown that levels in the blood do not exceed approximately 1 mg%, and levels in the urine are under 100 mg%; these levels are significantly less than the levels that prevailed when sulfadiazine was used for systemic therapy.

In order to determine localization of silver, studies were conducted with radioactive [110]AgSD (silver sulfadiazine) and these showed that the radioactive silver is localized in the burned skin and exudate with none absorbed or detected in the blood or the organs. In contrast, after therapy with soluble silver nitrate, low concentrations of silver were detected in the body fluids (22). This tissue localization frequently results in partial sterilization of the wound.

In contrast to these results, sulfamylon acetate is soluble and within a few hours the drug is completely absorbed and metabolized in the body to inactive products so that considerably higher doses are required to inhibit bacterial growth in the wounds. For this reason, dressings cannot be utilized because frequent reapplication of the sulfamylon acetate is required. The acetic acid portion of the drug causes metabolic acidosis and the mafenide portion is an inhibitor of carbonic anhydrase and induces the characteristic hyperventilation (1,5).

Because of the severe pain on application of sulfamylon acetate, essential alternate patient or double blind studies have been lacking. During the past year, however, Silvadene® was introduced into the Brooke Army Burn Center and compared carefully with sulfamylon. The results were presented in Toronto by Petersen, Pruitt et al. (23) and are decisive. In 144 patients treated with burns of over 30%, the gross survival in the sulfamylon patients was 22% in the 15- to 40-year age group with LA_{50} of 40%. Silver sulfadiazine treated patients in that same period had a gross survival of 55% in the same age group and a LA_{50} of 64.3%. Two other observations were made, the first was that the mean time of the death of patients treated with sulfamylon was 10 days while those treated with silver sulfadiazine was 28 days. The second observation was that 77% of the patients dying during silver sulfadiazine therapy had one or more positive blood cultures while only 30% of those dying during sulfamylon therapy had positive blood cultures, strongly suggesting that in the bulk of the sulfamylon treated patients, death resulted from something other than sepsis.

Another point of interest is the patients' bacteriological data; apparently, sulfamylon often better controlled the gram negative population of the burn wound with counts averaging 10^4 to 10^5. The major organisms in the sulfamylon treated patients were *Staphylococcus aureus* and *Candida albicans*. In contrast, the silver sulfadiazine treated patients routinely had quantitative counts of 10^7 organisms, primarily enterobacter. The fungal colonization was not seen with silver sulfadiazine but candida was a common occurrence in sulfamylon treated patients. In contrast to the application of sulfamylon, which is attended with a great deal of pain lasting as long as 30 minutes, silver sulfadiazine was not attended with pain and some patients requested application of the silver sulfadiazine to allay their pain. Early pulmonary problems were seen in 17 of the 40 patients (42%) treated with sulfamylon. [This is reminiscent of the findings of pulmonary hyaline membrane disease in animals by Ilahi (24)]. Their conclusion is that patients treated with silver sulfadiazine had a more benign clinical course than those treated with sulfamylon:

> "Finally and most important the earlier time of death, the more complex clinical course, the lower incidence of sepsis causing death in Sulfamylon treated patients all combine to strongly suggest the toxic effect of Sulfamylon when applied to a patient in the early post-burn period. It is our opinion that Sulfamylon should not be used on patients with greater than 30% total body surface burns in the immediate post-burn period" (23).

DATA ON DRUG SENSITIVITY

At this point a review of the frequency of drug sensitivity is relevant. Evidence of drug sensitivity was found in less than ten of more than 10,000 patients treated with silver sulfadiazine. The amino group of sulfamylon is separated from the benzene ring by a methyl group, and the resulting aliphatic amino differs greatly from the aromatic amino group of sulfonamides (25). The more basic aliphatic structure conveys a vastly greater incidence of sensitization and allergies. Patch tests showed that sulfonamides are only mild sensitizers while sulfamylon was a frequent offender. The allergic potency of sulfamylon is linked to the intramolecular distribution of charge, i.e., only an alkaline amino group makes the molecules act as an allergen. Sulfonamides do not react like sulfamylon and other aromatic *para*-amines (ethyl-amino-benzoates) and rarely give positive tests in patients.

A final point of comparison of these three drugs is the consideration that daily treatment of a burn surface of one square meter (which is equivalent to a 50% burn in an adult) requires 200 gm of silver nitrate (40 liters of 0.5% silver nitrate solution) or 26.6 gm of sulfamylon acetate (application of 500 gm of the cream twice daily with no dressings) or 4 gm of silver sulfadiazine (100 gm of Silvadene® cream) applied daily and usually covered with dressings.

CLINICAL RESULTS

There are reports from numerous burn units world wide which have confirmed the prophylactic and therapeutic efficacy of silver sulfadiazine. For example, Baxter (6) reported only 7 septic deaths in 315 patients (161 children and 157 adults under 70 years of age) with burns up to 60% of the body surface. Dickinson (7) had only 1 death among 40 children. In studies in which silver nitrate, silver sulfadiazine, mafenide, and other drugs were compared, Lowbury et al. (10) and MacMillan (3,8) reported a higher incidence of negative wound cultures, earlier skin grafting, and absence of pain on application of silver sulfadiazine. All clinicians observed healing of large areas initially thought to be full-thickness injury. Their experience, in addition to good control of infection, resulted frequently in delaying the decision to graft in many patients. In some instances, excessive delay in deciding to graft was detrimental in that contractures and scarring resulted. Wounds that do not show epithelial regeneration in 2–3 weeks should be grafted promptly. Other observations were a decreased need for systemic antibiotics, good nutrition, willingness to eat, and fewer supportive transfusions. Dickinson reported also the decreased need for hetero- or xenografts (7).

Certain questions remain unrsolved at this date; first and probably most important is the question as to the optimal frequency of application of the cream. Second is the relative advantages of the open and closed technique, the use of dressings, the frequency of tubbing, and the use of xeno-, hetero-, and autografts.

LOOKING AHEAD – ZINC SULFADIAZINE

In view of the highly satisfactory results obtained with silver sulfadiazine, research is continuing to improve topical therapy and one step in this direction is the synthesis and use of zinc sulfadiazine (26).

Wound healing, especially in burns, is a complex process for which zinc has been found essential by Prasad (27), Nielsen and associates (28), Henzel et al. (29), Larson and co-workers (30), and Brodribb and Ricketts (31). Burn patients in particular have poor appetites, lose weight, and often require zinc therapy and hyperalimentation as correlated by Cohen and associates (32). In an effort to obtain topical control of infection and simultaneously apply zinc for wound healing, zinc sulfadiazine was synthesized and investigated. Zinc, unlike silver, is a normal body constituent and the greater solubility of the zinc sulfadiazine in exudates can facilitate continuous replacement for the zinc reported lost after thermal or surgical trauma. Accordingly, silver and zinc sulfadiazine have been compared *in vitro* and in experimental burn wound sepsis (33). Comparison of several drugs is shown in Fig. 3. In numerous subsequent animal experiments zinc sulfadiazine proved highly effective in controlling pseudomonas infection in mice and in rats subjected to a thermal burn (26). Additional studies were carried out with the view to observing the effect of zinc sulfadiazine on wound healing. The animals with burns on the dorsum were retained for several weeks to evaluate the rate of healing and ultimate closure of the wound. In these experiments all untreated controls died in 7 to 10 days postburn, but all those treated survived and their wounds were measured (26). The measurements obtained by our method suggests that with daily application of zinc sulfadiazine, the wound closed sooner and healed more rapidly than with silver sulfadiazine.

A further step in the direction of improved therapy was the evaluation of combining one of the rare earth metals with silver sulfadiazine.

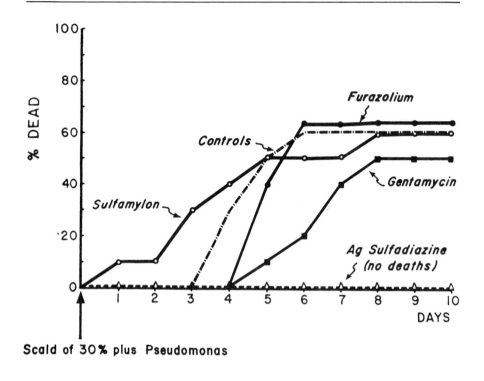

Scald of 30% plus Pseudomonas

3   Comparison of topical silver sulfadiazine and other drugs in controlling pseudomonas sepsis in mice scalded over 30% of body area. In numerous subsequent experiments, zinc sulfadiazine yielded equivalent or slightly better rates of survival (26).

In clinical studies, Monafo (34) reported that addition of cerium nitrate to Silvadene® enhanced the therapeutic effect of the Silvadene® in controlling infection in burn wounds. We then synthesized cerous sulfadiazine itself and conducted investigations of this new compound (35). The data, which at this point must be regarded as preliminary, indicates, that cerous sulfadiazine is a highly effective topical agent for control of pseudomonas infection. With cerous sulfadiazine in combination with silver sulfadiazine or with zinc sulfadiazine, or a combination of the three sulfadiazine compounds, improved therapeutic efficacy appears to be obtainable. Further studies and clinical trials are essential for final evaluation. These are now in progress.

COMPARISON OF MODE OF SILVER, ZINC, AND CERIUM SULFADIAZINE

As indicated above, the antimicrobial effect of silver sulfadiazine appears to result from the bonding of the silver by the paired bases of DNA (14,20). The mode of action of the zinc sulfadiazine is considerably different. Zinc sulfadiazine reacts with both DNA and RNA as described by Eichhorn and Butzow (36). In subsequent papers these authors investigated the interaction of zinc and other metal ions such as cerium with polynucleotides and observed that trivalent ions and, apparently, zinc degrade the polynucleotides (37). They found that unlike the bonding of silver to the paired bases of DNA, zinc and, presumably, cerium bond not only to the bases but attach also to the negative phosphate groups. Prolonged contact then induces degradation of the polynucleotides. Thus, their studies suggest a different mode of action for these new metal complexes of sulfadiazine. In this connection it should be noted that recent studies have described the interaction of amino acridines with DNA and suggest that this interaction is responsible for the antimicrobial effect of the potent amino acridine compounds (38). The point is that further study of the metal complexes of sulfonamides may be leading to new compounds which inhibit microbial growth by highly selective mechanisms unlike those described for other antimicrobial agents. These poorly soluble compounds remain in the wound for a long period of time and thereby inhibit microbial proliferation and eradicate bacteria from the wounds.

TOPICAL TREATMENT OF WOUNDS OTHER THAN BURNS WITH SILVER SULFADIAZINE

In view of the wide spectrum of antimicrobial activity of these compounds, their use for eradication of infection in wounds other than burns has been explored. Decubitus ulcers and chronic leg ulcers have healed rapidly with daily topical applications of Silvadene®. More extensive infections, such as laparotomy wounds with dehiscence and leakage of bowel contents from fistulae, have also been benefited. In vascular surgery, when a pseudomonas infection after an arterial graft

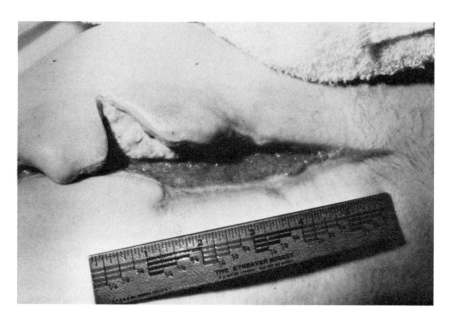

4

Pseudomonas infection in wound after femoral artery graft treated with AgSD.

threatened survival of the graft, the wound was opened and packed with Silvadene® daily. The extent of such a wound, from groin to ankle, is shown in Fig. 4 and the ultimate closure after one month of therapy is shown in Fig. 5. In children numerous pseudomonas dermal infections occurring during antileukemic therapy have been eradicated. In a limited number of adolescents, acne vulgaris has been treated successfully. Finally, in preliminary trials psoriatic lesions of the trunk and scalp have been benefited by daily use of zinc sulfadiazine applied topically.

In view of the efficacy against fungi and certain viruses, 3% silver sulfadiazine cream is under investigation for vaginal use. Preliminary trials have indicated relief of viral and fungal infections in the vaginal tract. In addition, the high potency against the gonococcus and *Treponema pallidum* suggests the usefulness of this cream for the prophylaxis and control of venereal disease. It should be emphasized that

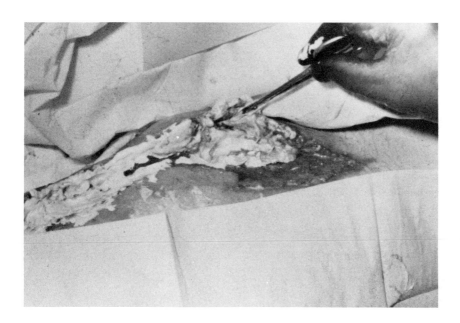

5   The same patient as in Fig. 4, 2 weeks later. Infection has been eradicated and healing has occurred.

these are merely suggested uses of these agents and that large numbers of careful clinical trials are essential for definitive evaluation.

SUMMARY

Silver sulfadiazine (Silvadene®, US; Flamazine, UK; Flammazine, Netherlands; Sulplata, South America) is proving to be a highly successful topical antimicrobial agent for control of burn wound infections. The advantages of a wide spectrum of activity, painless application, negligible toxicity, and ease of application contribute to the usefulness of this compound. These advantages have led to its use for wound infections other than burns, for skin ulceration, for certain dermatological lesions, and also for the prevention and treatment of various vaginal infections.

Described also are zinc sulfadiazine, which can provide zinc for wound healing, and cerous sulfadiazine, which contains the rare earth metal cerium. Their unique effects on cell biology may determine their specific roles in topical therapy.

ACKNOWLEDGMENT

Aided in part by the John A. Hartford Foundation and by Public Health Service research grant GM-18275 from the National Institute of General Medical Sciences.

REFERENCES

1. R.B. Lindberg, J.A. Moncrief. W.E. Switzer. The succesful control of burn wound sepsis. *J. Trauma* 5, 601–616 (1965).
2. C.L. Fox, Jr. (ed.). Early treatment of severe burns. *Ann. N.Y. Acad. Sci.* 150, 469–1012 (1968).
3. J.B. Lynch, S.R. Lewis (eds.). "Symposium on the Treatment of Burns," C.V. Mosby Co., St. Louis, 1973.
4. T.J. Krizek, M.C. Robson, R.C. Wray. Jr. Care of the burned patient in: "Management of Trauma" (W.R. Ballinger, R.B. Rutherford, G.D. Zuidema, eds.), 2nd ed. W.B. Saunders, Co., Philadelphia, pp. 650–718. 1973.
5. J.A. Moncrief. "Clinics in Plastic Surgery," W.B. Saunders. Co., Philadelphia, pp. 520–600. 1974.
6. C.R. Baxter. Topical use of 1.0% silver sulfadiazine, in: (H.C. Polk, Jr., and H.H. Stone, eds.) "Contemporary Burn Management," Little, Brown and Co., Boston, pp. 217–225. 1971.
7. S.J. Dickinson. Topical therapy of burns in children with silver sulfadiazine. *N.Y. State J. Med.* 73, 2045–2049 (1973).
8. R.P. Hummel, B. MacMillan, W.A. Altemeier. Topical and systemic antibacterial agents in the treatment of burns. *Ann. Surg.* 172, 370–384 (1970).
9. T.J. Krizek, D.V. Cossman. Experimental burn wound sepsis: Variations in response to topical agents. *J. Trauma* 12, 553–559 (1972).
10. E.J.L. Lowbury, D.M. Jackson, C.R. Ricketts, et al., Topical chemoprophylaxis for burns: Trials of creams containing silver sulfadiazine and trimethoprin. *Injury: Brit. J. Accident Surg.* 3, 18–24 (1971).
11. I.A. McDougall. Burns and the use of silver sulfadiazine *N.Z. J. Surg.* 42, 174–178 (1972).
12. J.N. Withers. Control of Pseudomonas infections in burns with silver sulfadiazine. *Hawaii Med. J.* 29, 298–300 (1970).
13. C.L. Fox, Jr. Silver sulfadiazine—A new topical therapy for Pseudomonas in burns. *Arch. Surg.* 96, 184–188 (1968).
14. C.L. Fox, Jr., B.W. Rappole, W. Stanford. Control of Pseudomonas in-

fection in burns by silver sulfadiazine. *Surg. Gyn. Obst.* 128, 1021–1026 (1969).

15. C.L. Fox, Jr. Use of silver sulfadiazine in burned patients, in: "Symposium on the Treatment of Burns" (J.B. Lynch, S.R. Lewis, eds.) C.B. Mosby Co., St. Louis, pp. 123–128 (1973).

16. J.R. Lloyd. Improved management of skin graft donor sites. *Arch. Surg.* 108, 561–565 (1974).

17. T. Tokumaru, Y. Shimizu, C.. Fox, Jr. Antiviral activities of silver sulfadiazine in ocular infection. *Res. Comm. Chem. Path. Pharmacol.* 8, 151–158 (1974).

18. T.J. Wlodrowski, H.S. Rosenkranz. Antifungal activity of silver sulfadiazine. *Lancet* 2, 739–740 (1973).

19. T.W. Chang, L. Weinstein. Inactivation of treponema pallidum by silver sulfadiazine. *Antimicrobial Agents Chemother.* 7, 538–539 (1975).

20a. S.M. Modak, C.L. Fox, Jr., Binding of silver sulfadiazine to the cellular components of Pseudomonas aeruginosa. *Biochem. Pharmacol.* 22, 2391–2404 (1973)

20b. C.L. Fox, Jr., S.M. Modak. Mechanism of silver sulfadiazine action on burn wound infections. *Antimicrobial Agents Chemother.* 5, 582–588 (1974).

21. J.D. Watson. "Molecular Biology of the Gene." p. 508. 1970. W.A. Benjamin, Co., New York.

22. W.W. Monafo, C.A. Moyer. The treatment of extensive thermal burns with 0.5% silver nitrate solution, in Early Treatment of Severe Burns. *Ann. N.Y. Acad. Sci.* 150, 937 (1968).

23. H.D. Peterson, B.A. Pruitt, A.D. Mason, et al. Prospective comparison of sulfamylon and silver sulfadiazine (in press).

24. M.A. Ilahi, J.B. Billote, A. Aoki, et al. Occurrence of pulmonary hyaline membrane disease in burned guinea pigs treated with topical sulfamylon. *Surg. Forum* 19, 64–66 (1968).

25. H.J. Bandmann, R. Breit. The mafenide story. *Brit. J. Derm.* 89, 219–221 (1973).

26. C.L. Fox, Jr., S.M. Modak, J.W. Stanford. Zinc sulfadiazine for topical therapy of Pseudomonas infection in burns. *Surg. Gyn. Obstet.* (in press).

27. A.S. Prasad. "Zinc Metabolism." Charles C. Thomas, Springfield, Ill., 1966.

28. S.P. Nielsen, B. Jemec. Zinc metabolism in patients with severe burns. *Scand. J. Plast. Reconstr. Surg.* 2, 47–52 (1968).

29. J.H. Henzel, M.S. DeWeese, E.L. Lighti. Zinc concentrations in healing wounds. *Arch. Surg.* 100, 349 (1970).

30. D.L. Larson, R. Maxwell, S. Abston, et al. Zinc deficiency in burned children. *Plast. Reconstr. Surg.* 46, 13-21 (1970).

31. A.J. Brodribb, C.R. Ricketts. Effects of zinc in healing of burns. *Injury*: *Brit. J. Accident Surg.* 3, 25 (1971).

32. I.K. Cohen, P.J. Schechter. Hypogeusia, anorexia, and altered zinc

metabolism following thermal burns. *J. Amer. Med. Assoc.* 223, 914–916 (1973).

33. C.L. Fox, Jr., A.C. Sampath, J.W. Stanford. Virulence of Pseudomonas infection of burned rats and mice—comparative efficacy of silver sulfadiazine and mafenide. *Arch. Surg.* 101, 508–512 (1970).

34. W.W. Monafo. Cerium nitrate—A new topical antiseptic for extensive burns. *Surgery* (in press).

35. C.L. Fox, Jr. Cerous sulfadiazine and its antimicrobial activity for the topical therapy of Pseudomonas infection in burn wounds (in press).

36. G.L. Eichhorn, J.J. Butzow. Interactions of metal ions with polynucleotides and related compounds. III. Degradation of polyribonucleotides by Lanthanum ions. *Biopolymers* 3, 79–94 (1965).

37. J.J. Butow, G.L. Eichhorn. Interactions of metal ions with polynucleotides and related compounds. IV. Degradation of polyribonucleotides by zinc and other divalent metal ions. *Biopolymers* 3, 95–107 (1965).

38. D.S. Drummond, F.W. Simpson-Gildemeister, A.R. Peacocke. Interaction of aminoacridines with deoxyribonucleic acid: effects of ionic strength, denaturation and structure. *Biopolymers* 3, 135–153 (1965).

39. R.H. Jensen, N. Davidson. Spectrophotometric, potentiometric, and density gradient ultracentrifugation studies of the binding of silver ion by DNA. *Biopolymers* 4, 17 (1966).

Transfer Factor for Candidiasis

CHARLES H. KIRKPATRICK

Our studies of patients with chronic mucocutaneous candidiasis was derived from an interest in abnormalities of cell-mediated immunity in man and their clinical consequences (1,2). However, before describing our investigations in these patients, I will briefly review our current understanding of the development of immunological competence and show how this model may be applied to clinical problems.

DEVELOPMENT OF THE IMMUNE RESPONSE

From studies in immunologically manipulated chickens, Cooper and co-workers (3) proposed the two-component model of development of immune competence. According to the model, bone marrow stem cells may receive differentiative influences from either of two sources: the thymus or the bursa of Fabricius. Thymus-dependent cells become "T" cells that respond to antigens by producing lymphokines (the effector molecules of cellular immunity) and are operative in immune responses such as delayed cutaneous hypersensitivity, allograft rejection, and graft vs. host reactions. On the other hand, cells that differentiate in the bursa

Table I. Serological Responses in Mucocutaneous Candidiasis

Test	Candidiasis patients	Control subjects
Candida agglutinins (serum)	17/20 > 1:128 10/20 > 1:512	≤1:128
Candida precipitins (serum)	17/20 positive	negative
Candida skin test (15 minutes)	25/27 positive	negative

become "B" cells which respond to antigens by synthesizing and secreting antibodies, the effector molecules of humoral immunity. The relative independence of these systems was shown by experiments in which newly-hatched chicks were thymectomized and irradiated several weeks prior to immunization. These birds developed normal antibody responses but had severely impaired cell-mediated immunity (3). Conversely, chicks that underwent bursectomy and irradiation and were later immunized had deficient antibody responses but were capable of developing normal cell-mediated immunity (3). Recent experiments have shown that the two systems are not totally independent. Thymus-derived cells (helper cells) are essential for optimal antibody responses to certain antigens (4), and other thymus-derived cells have suppressor activities and reduce the magnitude of antibody responses (5).

The relevance of the model to human diseases has been shown in patients with immune deficiency diseases. Children with congenital absence of the thymus have severely impaired cellular immunity but normal antibody responses; their lesion is functionally equivalent to the thymectomized-irradiated chickens. Patients with the x-linked form of congenital hypogammaglobulinemia have virtual absence of humoral immunity, yet most patients with this disorder develop delayed cutaneous hypersensitivity and reject skin grafts in a normal manner. Their immune deficiency is analogous to that seen in bursectomized-irradiated chicks. Other more complex immunodeficiencies apparently involve the stem cell populations.

It is within the general guidelines of this model that we have conducted the immunologic evaluations of the patients with chronic mucocutaneous candidiasis.

Table II. Delayed Cutaneous Hypersensitivity in Patients with
Chronic Mucocutaneous Candidiasis

Group	Response	Patients (No.)
I	No response to any antigen (anergy)	8
II	No response to candida — other responses such as SK-SD, mumps, or tetanus toxoid present	10
III	Response to candida present	9

IMMUNOLOGIC STUDIES IN CHRONIC MUCOCUTANEOUS CANDIDIASIS

Investigations of the serological responses by these patients have not revealed any deficiencies. Indeed, as shown in Table I, the antibody responses to candida antigens by candidiasis patients are often greater than the control subjects. These antibody responses probably involve all classes of immunoglobulins, and many patients with chronic mucocutaneous candidiasis have polyclonal hyperimmunoglobulinemia. Antibody responses to other antigens are usually normal.

A peculiar disorder that often accompanies chronic candidiasis is progressive endocrine failure that may affect multiple organs. Among our patients there are six patients with adrenal insufficiency, three patients with hypothyroidism and three patients with hypoparathyroidism. Antibodies against endocrine tissues are common in such patients (6,7), although it has not been established that they are involved in the pathogenesis of the endocrinopathies. Instead, they may reflect tissue injury caused by other mechanisms.

In contrast, studies of cell-mediated immune responses in patients with chronic mucocutaneous candidiasis have revealed multiple abnormalities. Assessment of these responses involves *in vivo* tests for delayed hypersensitivity to candida and other antigens and measurement of *in vitro* responses such as antigen-induced DNA synthesis and lymphokine production (1,8). It is essential to conduct both *in vivo* and *in vitro* tests to completely identify and characterize the immunological lesions in the patients.

Table II summarizes the delayed cutaneous hypersensitivity responses

Table III. Relationship of Age of Onset to Delayed Skin Responses

Age of onset	Complete anergy	Anergy to Candida	Responsive to Candida
≤ 3 years	8	7	2
>3 years	0	3	6

in our patients with candidiasis. Note that there are three patterns of responsiveness. One group was unresponsive to all of the antigens in the test panel. In the second group delayed reactions to Candida were not present, but the patients were capable of responding to other common antigens such as streptokinase–streptodornase (SK–SD), mumps skin test antigen, or tetanus toxoid. The patients in the third group developed normal delayed responses to Candida.

The relationship between the extent of the immunological defect and the age of onset of chronic mucocutaneous candidiasis is shown in Table III. Note that all of the anergic patients developed candidiasis during infancy or early childhood, while in most of the patients with positive skin tests the disease occurred later in life, usually near the end of the first decade or during adult years.

In vitro studies with blood lymphocytes from the candidiasis patients have provided additional evidence for the heterogeneity of immune deficiencies in these subjects. Table IV summarizes these results. Note that cells from the skin test-reactive patients responded to Candida antigens *in vitro* with increased DNA synthesis (lymphocyte transformation), and four of the six patients studied also made the lymphokine, migration inhibition factor (MIF).

Skin-test-negative patients were somewhat more heterogeneous in their *in vitro* responses. Five of the 18 skin-test-negative patients had normal lymphocyte transformation responses to stimulation with Candida; the remaining 13 patients were unresponsive in this test. Only one skin-test-negative patient produced MIF when his cells were exposed to Candida *in vitro*.

In summary, impaired reactivity to Candida antigens was present in 20 of the 26 patients described in Table IV.

Table IV. In Vitro Lymphocyte Responses in
Chronic Mucocutaneous Candidiasis

Patients with negative candida skin tests and:		18
1. Negative MIF* production (11 studied)	10	
2. Positive MIF production (11 studied)	1	
3. Negative lymphocyte transformation	13	
4. Positive lymphocyte transformation	5	
Patients with positive candida skin tests and:		8
1. Negative MIF production (6 studied)	2	
2. Positive MIF production (6 studied)	4	
3. Negative lymphocyte transformation	0	
4. Positive lymphocyte transformation	8	

*MIF = macrophage migration inhibition factor

THERAPEUTIC APPROACHES

In considering possible immunological measures for treating these patients, two questions were addressed. First, was it possible to correct the immunological lesion; and, second, would correction of the immunological defect be accompanied by any clinical benefits?

Our first approach to immunological therapy involved passive sensitization to candida antigens by transfusions of large numbers of immunocompetent cells from candida skin-test-positive, related, but genetically disparate donors (1,9). After the transfusions, the first patient, a 17-year-old-male, showed prompt conversion of delayed skin responses from negative to positive and his candida-stimulated lymphocytes made MIF (9). His mucocutaneous lesions slowly regressed and by 2 months were completely gone. About 6 months later the lesions recurred, and when he was restudied it was found that both his skin tests and MIF production had reverted to negative.

The second patient was a 25-year-old girl with minimal skin disease but extensive candidiasis of the mucous membranes. Following the cell transfusions, she, too, had a remission that lasted for 3 years during which she had a fullterm pregnancy without an exacerbation of candidiasis. Recently, she has again had episodes of oral and vaginal candidiasis.

These studies showed that the patients could develop immunological

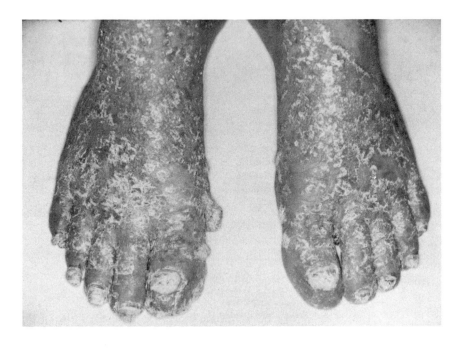

1 a.   (A) Mucocutaneous candidiasis of the feet prior to treatment with amphotericin B and transfer factor. (B) The same patient 3 years after amphotericin B therapy. The patient is receiving transfer factor every 4 months.

competence and that an immunotherapy program had therapeutic potential. However, viable cell transfusions were inconvenient and carried the risk of graft vs. host disease. We then elected to evaluate immunotherapy with transfer factor (10,11).

Six anergic patients with extensive mucocutaneous candidiasis were treated with monthly injections of transfer factor for 6 months. All other therapy was unchanged. All patients became skin-test positive to candida and other reactivities possessed by the transfer-factor donor. However, at the end of the 6-month trial, 4 patients were unchanged and 2 patients were worse. Thus, under the conditions employed in this trial, transfer factor in doses which caused conversion of delayed hypersensitivity was not an efficacious therapeutic agent.

The study design was then changed to include treatment of the

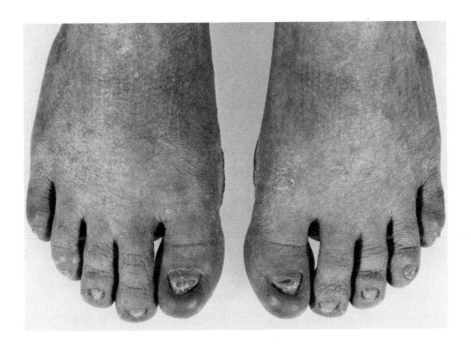

b.

patients with intravenous amphotericin B to induce remissions and to use transfer factor as a form of consolidation therapy. The total dose of amphotericin was 15–20 mg per/Kg and was given over 8–10 weeks (12). Near the end of this course, transfer factor was started. Doses were given monthly for 4 months and then less frequently; most patients are now receiving an injection every 4 months.

Currently, two patients are in cutaneous remissions 4 years after stopping amphotericin B (Fig. 1). Three other patients are in remissions after 3 years, 8 months, and 4 months, respectively. Thus, this protocol has been successful in controlling the cutaneous component of the disease.

The results with mucous membrane candidiasis have been less satisfactory. Both of our longest-treated patients have mild to moderate oral candidiasis that resists local therapy.

DISCUSSION AND CONCLUSIONS

Several conclusions may be drawn from the observations summarized in this paper. First, chronic mucocutaneous candidiasis is a heterogeneous disorder, both in its clinical presentations and in the associated immunological defects. In most studies, the immunologic lesions are limited to the thymus-dependent (T cell) system and are usually expressed as an inability of precursor T cells to respond to antigens by differentiating into effector cells. This is illustrated by the failure of antigen-stimulated cells to produce lymphokines and synthesize DNA. It should be noted that experiments by Rocklin (13) have suggested that lymphokine-producing cells and DNA-synthesizing cells are members of separate populations. The observations with candidiasis patients have further suggested that immunological lesions may affect both or either one of these cell lines.

The development basis for the immunological defect is unknown. Patients with candidiasis since infancy are often anergic and the defect may be congenital. The patients who develop candidiasis during adulthood are more perplexing. Some immunological data (12) suggest that patients have become tolerant to candida antigens as a consequence of chronic exposure, but this problem requires further study.

Transfer factor is a safe and effective agent for correcting the immunological lesions in candidiasis patients. However, in our experience it is of no clinical value unless used in conjunction with a systemic antibiotic such as amphotericin B. Its primary therapeutic effect appears to be prevention of relapses following amphotericin treatment. There are many unanswered questions concerning transfer factor. Aside from the unknown composition and mechanism(s) of action, there are practical problems such as specificity. These questions have not been addressed in our studies for two reasons: the rarity of normal transfer factor donors who do not have cellular immunity to candida and the paucity of patients who meet our immunological and clinical criteria for inclusion into the study. Obviously, additional studies must be done.

REFERENCES

1. C.H. Kirkpatrick, R.R. Rich, J.E. Bennett. Chronic mucocutaneous candidiasis-model-building in cellular immunity. *Ann. Intern. Med.* 74, 955–978 (1971).
2. C.H. Kirkpatrick. Immunology of chronic mucocutaneous candidiasis. *Derm. Dig.* 13, 15-21 (1974).

3. M.D. Cooper, D.Y. Perey, R.D.A. Peterson, A.E. Gabrielsen, R.A. Good. The two component concept of the lymphoid system. *Birth Defects Orig. Art. Ser.* 4, 7–12 (1968).
4. D.H. Katz, B. Benacerraf. The regulatory influence of activated T cells on B cell responses to antigen. *Adv. Immunol.* 15, 1–94 (1972).
5. R.K. Gershon, P. Cohen, R. Hencin, S.A. Liebhaber. Suppressor T cells. *J. Immunol.* 108, 586–595 (1972).
6. D.B. Louria, D. Shannon, G. Johnson, L. Caroline, A. Okas, C. Taschdjian. The susceptibility to moniliasis in children with endocrine hypofunction. *Trans. Assoc. Am. Physicians* 80, 236–248 (1967).
7. R.M. Blizzard, J.H. Gibbs. Candidiasis: studies pertaining to its association with endocrinopathies and pernicious anemia. *Pediatrics* 42, 231–237 (1968).
8. C.H. Kirkpatrick, R.R. Rich, T.K. Smith. Effect of transfer factor on lymphocyte function in anergic patients. *J. Clin. Invest.* 51, 2948–2958 (1972).
9. C.H. Kirkpatrick, R.R. Rich, R.G. Graw, T.K. Smith, I.D. Mickenberg, G.N. Rogentine. Treatment of chronic mucocutaneous moniliasis by immunologic reconstitution. *Clin. Exper. Immunol.* 9, 733–748 (1971).
10. H.S. Lawrence. Transfer factor. *Adv. Immunol.* 11, 195–266 (1969).
11. C.H. Kirkpatrick, J.I. Gallin. Treatment of infectious and neoplastic diseases with transfer factor. *Oncology* 29, 46–73 (1974).
12. C.H. Kirkpatrick, T.K. Smith. Chronic mucocutaneous candidiasis: immunologic and antibiotic therapy. *Ann. Intern. Med.* 80, 310–320 (1974).
13. R.E. Rocklin. Production of migration inhibitory factor by nondividing lymphocytes. *J. Immunol.* 110, 674–678 (1973).

Recent Advances in Dermatopharmacology

6

Transfer Factor Therapy of Infectious Diseases

DAVID A. STEVENS
and The Coccidioidomycosis
Cooperative Treatment Group

Transfer factor (TF) is an extract of disrupted leukocytes which has the capability of transferring the specific cell-mediated immunity of a donor to a recipient (1,2). The substance is apparently preformed within leukocytes and is released *in vitro* on exposure to antigen as early as 30–60 minutes after exposure. Evidence of transfer of cell-mediated immunity *in vivo* can be detected as early as 4 hours after injection, and the transfer can persist for over a year, even in the absence of exposure to antigen. Dr. Kirkpatrick has reviewed, earlier in this symposium, some of the basic properties of TF and its application to treatment of candidiasis. The following discussion will concern some clinical aspects of TF. Although the literature recognizes several different preparations, or "transfer factors", what follows concerns a dialyzable substance of <10,000 molecular weight.

It is of historical interest that studies with transfer of coccidioidin (an extract of the fungus *Coccidioides immitis*) reactivity demonstrated that transfer by TF could occur while boosting of latent reactivity in the recipient could be almost completely excluded as the mechanism of TF action. This was done by transfer experiments using coccidioidin-

Table I. Summary of Immunotherapeutic Attempts[a]

Therapy	Result on immunological parameters
One unit of whole blood	None
Transfer factor #1 (1.75 ml)[b]	Conversion to PPD skin-test positivity
Transfer factor #2 (3.0 ml)	Conversion to spherulin skin-test posi-·tivity, temporary conversion to coc-cidioidin skin-test positivity
Transfer factor #3 (2.83 ml)	No additional reactivity conferred
Buffy coats from four units of blood	Temporary boosting of spherulin positivity

[a]Reprinted with permission from *Cellular Immunology* (5)
[b]Volume of packed leukocytes used to prepare transfer factor.

negative recipients who had never visited *C. immitis* endemic areas (3).

In addition to potential applications to candidiasis, in passing we should mention studies on leprosy. In the lepromatous form of the disease, TF therapy has resulted in skin test conversions, reactive changes in skin infiltrates, and even erythema nodosum (presumably a manifestation of hyperreactivity) (4).

Studies of TF in coccidioidomycosis are important, even though many practitioners may never see a case, because they are an example of what may be possible with this approach in mycotic infections, i.e., it is a model. Many patients with disseminated coccidioidomycosis have cutaneous anergy to coccidioidin (recent analyses indicate ¾ of patients with disseminated or progressive disease are anergic), and many have deficient immune responses as assayed *in vitro*. Two-thirds of such patients don't have a blastogenic lymphocyte response to coccidioidin *in vitro*, and ¾ fail to produce the lymphokine migration inhibitory factor (MIF). In most of these patients the defect is selective—they respond normally to nonspecific mitogens and to other antigens but not to the one present in large amounts in their bodies. Anergy in these forms of the disease is predictive in that it is associated with fatal progression. Likewise, spontaneous or antibiotic therapy-related recovery of cell-mediated immunity is associated with remissions. Attempts to boost cell-mediated immunity are therefore logical, particularly since the disease is often resistant to the currently available therapy, amphotericin B.

An example of therapeutic efforts with TF in this disease is the patient we reported (5) with recurrent pulmonary coccidioidomycosis. She had four reactivations of her disease, each leading to a cavity. She

Table II. Members of the Coccidioidomycosis Cooperative
Treatment Group (CCTG)

Arizona	Texas
Phoenix	University of Texas at San Antonio
Dr. Bernard Levine	Dr. David Drutz
	Dr. Richard Graybill
California	Dr. Daniel Thor
University of California	San Antonio State Chest Hospital
Davis	Dr. Joseph Vivas
Dr. Demosthenes Pappagianis	Dr. Rebecca Cox
San Diego	
Dr. Antonino Catanzaro	
Dr. Kenneth Moser	
San Francisco	
Dr. Lynn Spitler	
Stanford	
Dr. David Stevens	
Bakersfield	
Dr. Hans Einstein	
Fresno	
Dr. Robert Libke	

had a selective immune defect as described above. Immune reconstitution was attempted five times, as shown in Table I. Whereas whole blood
from a coccidioidin-positive donor failed to affect any immunological
parameter, the first dose of TF converted her response to PPD (the
donor was PPD-positive) but not to the *C. immitis* antigens. A larger
dose of TF did succeed in this. The responsiveness to *C. immitis* antigens
was seen best with spherulin, a new reagent derived by Dr. H.B. Levine
from the spherule phase of the fungus, which we have been studying for
about 3 years (6-9). Our studies indicate this is a more sensitive probe
of cellular immunity than coccidioidin. In conjunction with these immunological changes, her disease stabilized.

Similar and more impressive clinical responses have been seen in
association with such immunotherapeutic attempts by several workers
(10-13). Because of the clinical variability of these diseases, and the
lack of standardized reagents, definite cause and effect relationships
cannot be established by such approaches or by any one team. Therefore a number of investigators have banded together in hopes of developing a controlled trial of TF in this disease. We call ourselves the
Coccidioidomycosis Cooperative Treatment Group and include the
groups indicated in Table II.

Table III. Immunological Changes Following Transfer Factor

	Total number of patients	Number with positive pre transfer factor	Number converting post transfer factor
Skin test	44	8	24
Blastogenesis	32	9	18
MIF	28	3	21

Table III shows the results of immunological evaluations performed by this group on patients with disseminated or progressive pulmonary coccidioidomycosis studied to date, in advance of a randomized trial. This was compiled for us recently by Dr. Graybill (14). Though most of these patients had been followed for a long time before TF was administered and were known to be anergic, thus lessening the likelihood that the conversions are spontaneous, the timing of the conversions also indicates the conversions were due to TF. Conversions demonstrated on retests within 10 days after TF are almost certainly, and those beyond 10 days still highly likely, due to the TF (Table IV).

Table V shows the clinical results of the nonrandomized studies to date. Three-fifths of the group clinically improved, despite the advanced nature of most of these cases and their refractoriness to conventional therapy. Evidence has already been obtained from these studies that repeated therapy with TF may be needed. These results encourage us to continue to try to advance towards a cooperative randomized clinical trial. We solicit referral of suitable cases and hope to define the role of TF in this disease in a double-blind crossover study. One set of standardized pretested reagents will be used. Patients will receive multiple doses. Serial immunological observations will be made. Defined and standardized criteria of improvement will be employed. The patients will be stratified into groups by various criteria, including race, sex, age, organ involvement, duration of disease, immune defects, and prior therapy. We would like to compare TF prepared from a coccidioidin-positive donor with a placebo and with TF prepared from a coccidioidin-negative donor. The reason for the latter is the suggestion from some quarters that TF may act as a nonspecific booster.

The importance of such a controlled, randomized approach was brought home to us in a study we performed on the effect of TF therapy on warts (15). This is the first randomized, double-blind study of TF

Table IV. Time of *In Vitro* or *in Vivo* Conversion

	Duration between pre/post studies			
Neg → Pos	<4 Days	4-10 Days	>10 Days	Total
Converted one or more tests	7	5	10	22
No conversions	3	3	8	14
Total	10	8	18	36

Table V. Clinical Improvement Following Transfer Factor in 49 Patients

None	Modest/Gradual	Dramatic
19	18	12

that I'm aware of. There is much evidence that an immune response is the control mechanism in warts. This evidence includes histological studies and a variety of immunological studies, which are reviewed elsewhere (15,16).

Our general plan was to record the sites involved with warts, and the number and size of warts at each site. Three observers rated the patients as worse, no change (0), partial remission (+), or complete remission (+ +) at each site and overall. The patients were given an initial test dose of TF corresponding to 10^7 disrupted leukocytes. As no patients developed adverse reactions, a second dose of the equivalent of 10^8 leukocytes was given 1 week later. Two weeks later a final dose equal to 10^8 leucocytes was given. The patients were observed a total of 7 weeks.

The genesis of the study was that after reports of TF therapeutic efficaciousness in the Wiskott–Aldrich syndrome appeared (2), a series of patients were started on treatment at Stanford Children's Hospital. One such 2-year-old patient with multiple warts developed erythema at all wart sites after a dose of TF, and in 1–2 weeks his warts regressed completely. The donor was questioned, and he had had spontaneous regression at multiple warty sites 6–12 months previously. A pilot study

Table VI. Therapeutic Result in Transfer Factor- and
Placebo-Treated Groups[a]

Observer rating[b]	Number of patients[c]	
	Transfer factor	Placebo
0,0,0	5	8
0,0,+	1	3
0,+,+	1	0
+,+,+	1	1
+,+,++	1	2
+,++,++	1	1
++,++,++	2	1

[a]Reprinted with permission from *Clinical and Experimental Immunology* (15).

[b]Ranking by three independent observers is shown. 0, no change; +, partial remission; ++, complete remission. (e.g., 0, 0, +, two observers rated the patients' disease as showing no overall change and the other indicated a partial remission.)

[c]Not shown are two patients who were not seen at the final visit by one observer. One patient given transfer factor was rated +, + by two observers and one patient given placebo was rated +, ++ by two observers.

with six patients was initiated, and three completed the study. Two patients had partial regression after the second dose and complete regression after the third, and the other had complete regression at two of three sites. Of the three lost to followup during the study, one had partial regression at some sites and complete regression at others.

We then initiated a randomized double-blind study. In it, some dramatic responses were seen, including complete remissions in the first weeks of study. At the end of the study, the code was broken. Table VI shows the results. As you can see, there was no difference between the two groups. There were complete and partial remissions in both groups. The six dramatic responses were evenly divided between both groups. There was excellent agreement between all three observers. Of 28 patients rated by all three observers, 18 were scored identically. Two of the three observers were in agreement for all patients, and no patient was rated more than one category higher or lower than any other observer.

The patients were also divided by several variables, including sex, disease extent (mild, moderate, and severe by number, size, and number of areas of warts), prior therapy, body surface area, and each observer's independent evaluations, into sets of subgroups. There was no evidence of a trend toward statistical significance in any subgroup.

The greatest difficulty in interpretation of these negative results is the lack of another test of competence of the TF preparation. The donor didn't have any unusual antigen reactivity that could be used as a marker. The same preparations were used in treatment of a series of Wiskott–Aldrich patients, and the investigators doing that study felt their results confirmed the reports in the literature. A high rate of spontaneous regressions could also explain an inability to show differences between TF and placebo. There is some evidence that humoral rather than cellular immunity may be related to regressions of warts. TF would not be expected to alter humoral immunity. It is possible that patients with immune deficiencies are responsive to lower doses of TF than healthy individuals. Finally, bigger doses of TF may produce a different result. A dose equivalent to 8.5×10^7 leukocytes is the minimum dose needed for systemic transfer. Our total dose corresponded to 2.1×10^8 cells, but more may be needed for therapy than is needed for transfer of skin test reactivity.

In any case, this experience must serve as a caution for claims of efficacy of TF in uncontrolled situations, especially where the natural history of the disease being treated is variable. Other modalities of treatment for warts need to be tested in a similar, controlled fashion.

ACKNOWELDGMENTS

Supported by grants from the American Lung Association and the Brown-Hazen Fund.

REFERENCES

1. H.S. Lawrence and F.T. Valentine, Transfer factor and other mediators of cellular immunity. *Amer. J. Path.* 60, 437–450 (1970).
2. A.S. Levin, *et al.*, Transfer factor therapy in immune deficiency states. *Ann. Rev. Med.* 24, 175–208 (1973).
3. F.T. Rapaport, *et al.*, Transfer of delayed hypersensitivity to coccidioidin in man. *J. Immunol.* 84: 358–367 (1960).
4. W.E. Bullock, *et al.*, An evaluation of transfer factor as immunotherapy for patients with lepromatous leprosy. *N. Eng. J. Med.* 287, 1053–1059 (1972).
5. D.A. Stevens, *et al.*, Immunotherapy in recurrent coccidioidomycosis. *Cell Immunol.* 12, 37–48 (1974).

6. D.A. Stevens, *et al.*, Dermal sensitivity to different doses of spherulin and coccidioidin. *Chest.* 65, 530–533 (1974).

7. S.C. Deresinski, *et al.*, Soluble antigens of mycelia and spherules in the *in vitro* detection of immunity to Coccidioides immitis. *Infect. Immun.* 10, 700–704 (1974).

8. D.A. Stevens. *et al.*, Spherulin in clinical coccidioidomycosis. *Chest* 68, 697–702 (1975).

9. H.B. Levine, *et al.* Spherulin and coccidioidin: cross reactions in dermal sensitivity to histoplasmin and paracoccidioidin. *Amer. J. Epid.* 101, 512–516 (1975).

10. J.R. Graybill, *et al.*, Immunologic and clinical improvement of progressive coccidioidomycosis following administration of transfer factor. *Cell. Immunol.* 8, 120–135 (1973).

11. P. Cloninger, *et al.*, Immunotherapy with transfer factor in disseminated coccidioidal osteomyelitis and arthritis. *West. J. Med.* 120, 322–325 (1974).

12. A. Catanzero, *et al.*, Immunotherapy of coccidioidomycosis. *J. Clin. Invest.* 54, 690–701 (1974).

13. D.A. Stevens, Transfer factor: treatment in coccidioidomycosis. Third International Symposium on Mycoses, *Pan American Health Organization* 304, 72–79 (1975).

14. J.R. Graybill, *et al.*, Transfer factor in coccidioidomycosis. *Clin. Res.* 23, 304 (1975).

15. D.A. Stevens, *et al.*, Randomized trial of transfer factor treatment of human warts. *Clin. Exp. Immunol.* 21, 520–524 (1975).

16. K.E.K. Rowson and B.W.J. Mahy. Human papova (wart) virus. *Bacteriol. Rev.* 31, 110–131 (1967).

Recent Advances in Dermatopharmacology

7

An Overview of Corticosteroid-Antibiotic Preparations

C. CARNOT EVANS

Combination products have been used by dermatologists for generations. Many of us have added some salicylic acid or tar to a formulation to achieve a desired therapeutic effect. It was only a few short years ago when the compounding of creams and ointments was jealously guarded. With each change in the formulation it was anticipated that there would be greater patient acceptance and greater effectiveness for the condition being treated.

As pharmaceutical firms began producing more dermatological products, it was only natural that they become interested in developing products containing more than one ingredient. There was a ready market in dermatologists who had been using such products. With such a wealth of ingredients to choose from, it was not surprising that a barrage of topical combination drugs became marketed. Along with this came expanded claims which were increased wth each ingredient that was added to the product.

In the mid-1960's, the National Academy of Sciences/National Research Council was asked to review the efficacy of all drugs marketed between 1938 and 1962. They created a number of panels that included all of the medical specialities. In their review of fixed combinations, only 45 of some 1200 were rated as effective. The remainder were rated as "ineffective" or "effective, but," meaning that the product itself was effective but that not all the ingredients were needed to produce the claimed effect.

The Food and Drug Administration (FDA) acted upon the panel recommendations and in the late 60's began legal proceedings to remove certain combination drugs from the market, among them some of the most widely used products in the nation. The pioneering legal case, from the standpoint of the agency, was the Pan-Alba decision of October 20, 1970. As a result of this court decision, the combination of tetracycline and novobiocin was removed from the market for lack of safety and lack of evidence that both components contributed to the drug product's effect.

The present Food and Drug Administration policy for fixed-combination prescription drugs was published in the Federal Register on October 15, 1971. It was developed in consultation with leaders in clinical pharmacology and medicine and was finalized after broad input from the medical profession, many scientific societies, the pharmaceutical industry, and the public. In spite of this wide knowledge of the conditions under which the Food and Drug Administration is prepared to approve fixed combinations, there has been concern on the part of many physicians and the drug industry that all combination products are to be removed from the market. The Food and Drug Administration combination policy is an expression of medical rationality not of anticombination prejudice. It is also a logical application of the legal requirements of the Food, Drug and Cosmetic Act to fixed-combination drugs.

The fixed-combination policy for prescription drugs sets out two fundamental requirements for an approvable combination: (1) Each component must make a contribution to the claimed effect, or one component must enhance the safety of the principal active ingredient, and (2) the dosage of each component must be such that the combination is safe and effective for significant patient populations requiring concurrent therapy as defined in the labeling for the drug. Our basic position is based on the concept that all drugs are to some degree potentially hazardous and should not be taken if they are not needed. The need for evidence that both components of a combination contribute to the claimed effect is implicit in the efficacy requirements of the Food, Drug and Cosmetic Act. This requirement was embodied in the New Drug Regulations, even before the 1971 publication of the combination policy. The regulations state "An application for a combination drug may be refused unless there is substantial evidence that each ingredient designated as active makes a contribution to the total effect claimed for the drug combination."

This requirement that both components contribute to the claimed effect has been the basis for disapproving a number of fixed combination products. Among the products disapproved to date are some old drugs and tonics of bizarre composition, but also among them are some of the most popular remedies in the land, such as several antibiotic combinations, erythromycin–sulfonamide combinations, steroid–aspirin combinations, and steroid–antihistamine combinations.

It should also be emphasized that some combinations have been able to satisfy the requirement that both components contribute to the claimed effect, for example, ampicillin–probenecid for gonorrhea, trimethoprim–sulfamethoxazole for recurrent urinary tract infections, estrogen–progestogen for contraception, and thiazide–reserpine for hypertension.

Three panels of dermatologists evaluated the dermatological drugs in the National Academy of Science (NAS) Review. They were supplied with all of the available background data on the individual drugs and the combinations. All of the steroid–antibiotic topicals were rated "less than effective."

A typical drug in this group was a hydrocortisone–neomycin combination recommended for atopic eczema, neurodermatitis, nummular eczema, food eczema, contact dermatitis, anogenital pruritus, stasis dermatitis, and to prevent or eradicate secondary bacterial complications. The panel evaluated this product as "Effective, but . . . " with the following comments:

> "The Panel believes that these conditions are responsive to the incorporated steroid alone, even in the presence of low grade secondary infection. In the event of significant bacterial infection systemic antibiotics should be used. The additional topical antibiotics exposes the patient to possible sensitivity reactions. The Panel suggests that the company document the superiority of the combination. Furthermore, the Panel is not aware of any proven prophylactic value of this preparation against infection in these dermatoses."

The second indication recommended for this product was "treatment of superficial infections of the skin amenable to neomycin therapy." The panel evaluated this claim as possibly effective and they had the following comment: "The Panel believes that as pyodermas need antimicrobial therapy they are best treated by the appropriate systemic antibiotic." As an additional comment the panel stated that "the labeling for these products should clearly indicate that neomycin is a cutaneous sensitizer"

The agency has concurred with the judgment of these distinguished panel members. We recognize that topical steroids are effective in many dermatoses. When the dermatoses are complicated by infection it is possible that the infected dermatoses will respond more satisfactorily to a combination of a corticosteroid and an appropriate topical antibiotic. Further study is needed, however, to demonstrate that the topical antiinfective-steroid combinations are in fact more effective than the individual components.

It may be appropriate at this point to note that topical antibiotics along with other topical antimicrobials are under exaluation by the Antimicrobial II Panel of the OTC Review. This is an extension of the panel that reviewed hexachlorophene and the antibacterial soaps. It consists of seven members, including two dermatologists.

In their preliminary review they have not placed a single topical antibiotic in the "generally recognized as safe and effective" group for skin infections. This includes well known drugs such as neomycin, polymyxin, bacitracin, gramicidin, and tetracycline. Their current position is that there is insufficient documentation that these antibiotics are effective, and more study is needed. This supports the position originally taken by the panels under the National Academy of Sciences Review.

Under the terms of a decision by the U.S. Court of Appeals for the District of Columbia, drugs rated "possibly effective" were to have been dealt with by the agency in mid-1974. We concluded, however, that this group of drugs had not been adequately studied and might fill a valid medical need and that more time should be permitted for studying them. Accoringly, in the Federal Register of October 9, 1974, we requested that manufacturers submit studies which could provide data on steroid–antibiotic combinations and in particular could demonstrate the contribution of the antibiotic.

Further problems present themselves, however. Many firms manufacture different dosage forms such as the cream, ointment, spray, etc. If one dosage form is shown to be effective, can other forms and concentrations be considered effective, or must this also be shown by controlled studies? How can we be assured of a product's effectiveness with the least effort and the least taxation of resources available for drug testing,

The making of regulatory judgments on combination products is an exercise in logic, requiring knowledge of the law, FDA policy, and the clinical data on the drug. We cannot base our judgments upon the fact that a combination is popular in medical practice or has been in use for many years but must rely on scientific data which meets exacting standards.

We all know that some combinations are useful and important in the practice of medicine. We also know that some offer no advantages in effectiveness or safety over their major active ingredient. Our job is to identify the products which are effective and pick them out from the hundreds of fixed combinations on the market. A major part of that job is working with investigators and manufacturers to determine the kinds of studies needed and the deficiencies in the present studies In the end we hope to provide assurance to physicians that any combination drug on the market is effective for its indicated uses and that all components contribute to the effect.

I can assure you that the FDA staff is very conscious of its responsibilities in decision making on combination drugs. We welcome comments from members of the National Program for Dermatology and other interested parties. We appreciate the opportunity to present our views to you on this important subject.

Recent Advances in Dermatopharmacology

8

A Cooperative Double-Blind Study of an Antibiotic/Corticoid Combination in Impetiginized Atopic Dermatitis

GERALD N. WACHS

INTRODUCTION

Dermatological opinion is divided on the question of whether to use an antibiotic/steroid combination or a corticoid alone, in the topical treatment of steroid-responsive dermatoses evidencing signs of infection. Blank (1), Davis (2), Larsen (3), and others suggest that corticoids alone can be used in the treatment of impetiginized dermatoses. On the other hand, there are many dermatologists who feel that the advantages of adding an antibiotic to a topical corticoid outweigh the risks of sensitization (4–13). Most likely, each member of the audience today would fall into one of these two groups.

A particularly significant contribution to the discussion of this problem is the recent communication by Leyden, Marples, and Kligman (14) in which they describe recovery of high concentrations of staph. aureus in lesions of atopic dermatitis even in the absence of clinical signs of infection. They suggest that high numbers of *Staphylococcus aureus* may aggravate the underlying lesion. Blank has also suggested this as a result of his studies.

Table I. Investigators and Their Contributions
to the Study Population

Investigator	BV/G	BV	G
Dr. Bender (Conn.)	2	3	2
Dr. Bluefarb (Ill.)	1	2	2
Dr. Cohen (N.Y.)	6	5	7
Dr. Dickey (Pa.)	2	2	2
Dr. Frost (Fla.)	1	3	0
Dr. Kenney (Wash., D.C.)	0	1	0
Dr. Levy (Calif.)	0	1	1
Dr. McCleary (Calif.)	1	1	0
Dr. Pass (N.Y.)	2	2	3
Dr. Rosenberg (Tenn.)	5	4	5
Dr. Smith, J.G. (Ga.)	1	1	1
Dr. Spencer (Ill.)	4	2	4
Total	25	27	27

The present communication reports a cooperative controlled double-blind study of the therapeutic effects of a fixed combination gentamicin betamethasone valerate cream preparation compared with each of its ingredients alone in the treatment of infected atopic dermatitis.* Twelve physician investigators took part in the study. (Table I).

A double-blind study of 79 patients with impetiginized atopic dermatitis is reported. Eighteen (72%) of 25 patients treated with a fixed-combination cream containing gentamicin 0.1% and betamethasone valerate 0.1% were judged to have an excellent response to therapy, compared with 15 (56%) of 27 treated with the corticoid alone and 8 (30%) of 27 treated with the topical antibiotic agent alone. Results, while not conclusive, suggest that combination therapy is the most effective way to treat impetiginized atopic dermatitis and that a larger study might provide even more clear-cut evidence.

METHODS AND MATERIALS

A randomized double-blind technique was employed, the usual precautions being observed with respect to preserving the "blinding"

---

* The Schering Corporation does not intend to market this preparation in the United States. The study is reported as a contribution to a better understanding of the problem under discussion.

of both patients and therapists. To aid in achieving uniformity in diagnosis and in grading of responses to treatment, the investigators assembled for study and discussion of Kodachrome slides illustrating the pre- and posttreatment appearance of lesions of infected atopic dermatitis. As they sat around the room each investigator rated each patient. It was amazing how uniform the ratings were as evaluated by the individual investigators. They seldom varied by more than one grade. Data was recorded on a standardized case record form.

Each physician agreed to attempt to empanel 15 patients, with no restrictions as to the race and sex of patients. No pregnant patients, no children under one year of age, and no patients with known renal disease were accepted, nor were patients with initial symptoms severe enough to warrant the use of systemic antibiotics. For patients receiving a systemic antibiotic or corticoid at the time of selection for the study, a three-week drug-free "wash-out" period was required; for those receiving prior topical therapy, one week without treatment.

Patients under the care of an individual investigator were randomly assigned in such a way that five were to receive the plain antibiotic, five the plain steroid, and five the combination cream. Medication was applied three times daily and no occlusive dressings were used. Patients were required to abstain from the use of medicated soaps throughout the period of study. No other systemic or topical antibiotics, corticoids, or antihistamines were permitted in the care of these patients; those for whom such treatment became necessary were considered "treatment failures."

Specimens for culture and sensitivity were obtained prior to treatment, on the eighth day and again on the twenty-second day. The cultures were performed on conventional media, i.e., TSA blood agar and thioglycollate broth. For measurement of antibiotic sensitivity the disc method of Kirby–Bauer was used. A urinalysis was performed at every visit.

In an attempt to quantify a subjective evaluation each investigator graded the following at each visit: (1) An overall or "global" assessment of the condition, overall severity; (2) Degree of inflammation; (3) Degree of infection.

Additionally, the following list of signs and symptoms was graded: erythema, pruritus, pustules, crusting, exudation, vesiculation, and lichenification. Investigators were required to grade each patient with respect to each symptom at each visit, according to the rating scale shown (Table II).

In order to be accepted for the study, a clear clinical diagnosis of infected atopic dermatitis had to be established with an initial overall

Table II. Rating Scale for Signs and Symptoms

Score	Interpretation
0	Complete absence
1	
2	Slight
3	
4	Mild to moderate
5	
6	Moderate to severe
7	
8	Severe
9	
10	Very severe-worst case ever seen

Table III. Grading Scheme for Final Evaluation of Response to Treatment

Score	Results
Excellent	Complete clinical control of condition (75% or better)
Good	Moderate clinical control of condition (50% - 75%)
Fair	Partial control of condition (25% - 49%)
Poor	Less than 25% improvement, or a worsening of the condition

rating of 5 or higher ("moderate to severe"). Follow-up visits were scheduled for the fourth, eighth, fifteenth, and twenty-second days of treatment. At each follow-up visit in addition to the evaluations previously described the investigators also rated the results of treatment. Finally, at the conclusion of the treatment period, an overall evaluation of each patient's response to treatment was made, as shown in Table III.

Table IV. Mean Statistical Differences: Corticoid,
Antibiotic, Corticoid/Antibiotic
All Investigators[a]

	BV/G	BV	G[b]
Degree of infection			
Initial	5.1	5.0	5.5
Final	0.0	1.4	1.8
Degree of inflammation			
Initial	5.8	5.9	6.2
Final	0.7	1.4	3.8
Overall evaluation of severity of condition			
Initial	6.1	6.1	6.6
Final	1.0	1.8	4.2

[a]Eleven point scale where 0 = none and 10 = very severe.
[b]Patient 4: Dr. Bender, omitted – no responses for final visit.

RESULTS

A total of 83 patients were enrolled, of which 79 were considered acceptable. There were 4 dropouts. Twenty-five patients were treated with the combination preparation, 27 received only betamethasone valerate and 27 received only gentamicin.

As indicated in Table IV, combination therapy reduced the mean scores for infection, inflammation, and overall severity of the 79 patients from the initial range of 5.1–6.1 down to the range of 0.00–1.0, while each of the two agents, given alone, had a less marked effect. Analyses of variance of these data yield probabilities which in most, but not all cases are significant. (Table V). No initial differences were found.

All patients enrolled were clinically judged to have moderate to severe impetiginized atopic dermatitis. Nevertheless, not all the initial cultures demonstrated the presence of bacteria and not all the species identified are customarily regarded as pathogens in otherwise uncomplicated dermatoses. A list of organisms found on initial culture is shown in Table VI. Evaluation of the culture results shows how accurate the clinicians were in their original diagnosis of infection.

Table V. Probabilities Associated with Treatment Differences
(Infection, Inflammation, Overall Severity)

	Rx-BV/G vs. Rx-BV	Rx-BV/G vs. Rx-G
Degree of infection	$p > 0.05$	$p < 0.01$
Degree of inflamation	$p > 0.20$	$p < 0.01$
Overall severity	$p > 0.20$	$p < 0.01$

Table VI. Bacteriological Data on Initial Cultures

Organism	Combination therapy	Betamethasone	Gentamicin	Total
Proteus spp.	–	–	1	1
Pseudomonas spp.	1	–	–	1
Staphylococcus spp.	21	20	22	63
Beta-hemolytic Strep	–	2	–	2
No Growth	–	–	1	1
Nonpathogens[a]	3	5	3	11
Totals	25	27	27	79

[a]The following organisms were cultured and were judged not to be pathogenic: Alcaligines, *B. subtilis, E. coli,* diphtheroids, Enterococcus, Herellia, Klebsiella, *Staph glococcus, albus* and *staphyloepidermis,* and various species of Streptococcus other than beta-hemolytic species.

From a purely bacteriological point of view, and without regard to the clinically judged outcomes of treatment, it is of some interest to pursue the matter of changes in the results of cultures with treatment. Data bearing on this point are presented. For each treatment, the results of initial cultures are tabulated against the results of final cultures (Table VII).

Of 25 patients treated with the combination cream, (Rx-BV/G), 22 initially cultured a pathogen. After 3 weeks, 23 patients had a final culture; only 6 remained positive.

Table VII. Outcome of Treatment
Initial Cutlure vs. Final Culture for Specific Pathogenic

Initial	Proteus	Pseudomona	Streptococcus Coag (+)	Streptococcus Coag (−)	Not done	No growth	Nonpathogen	Totals
Rx BV/G								
Pseudomonas species	—	—	—	—	—	1	—	1
Staphylococcus aureus coag (+)	—	—	4	—	1	5	3	13
Staphylococcus aureus coag (−)	—	—	—	2	1	4	1	8
Nonpathogens	—	—	—	—	—	1	2	3
Subtotal	—	—	4	2	2	11	6	25
Rx-BV								
Staphylococcus aureus coag (+)	1	—	3	1	1	3	3	12
Staphylococcus aureus coag (−)	—	—	—	3	1	2	2	8
Beta-hemolytic streptococcus	—	—	1	—	1	—	—	2
Nonpathogen	—	1	—	—	—	3	1	5
Subtotal	1	1	4	4	3	8	6	27
Rx-G								
Proteus species	—	—	—	—	—	1	—	1
Staphylococcus aureus coag (+)	—	1	4	—	4	2	3	15
Staphylococcus aureus coag (−)	—	—	—	—	—	1	6	7
No growth	—	—	—	—	—	1	—	1
Nonpathogen	—	—	—	—	1	1	1	3
Subtotal	—	1	4	—	6	6	10	27
Totals	1	2	12	6	11	25	22	79

Of the 27 patients treated with plain corticoid, (Rx-BV), 22 cultures initially demonstrated the presence of a skin pathogen. After 3 weeks of treatment, 24 patients were recultured; 10 pathogens were identified. (One of the final culture pathogens was recovered from a patient whose initial culture was nonpathogenic).

Of the 27 treated with gentamicin alone, (Rx-G), 23 initially cultured a pathogen. After 3 weeks, 21 patients had a final culture. Five were still positive for pathogens.

Pairwise comparison of these data using the Fisher Exact Probability Test demonstrates that the number of remaining pathogens in each of the 3 treatment groups is not significant ($p > 0.30$). It is of interest to note, however, that the plain corticoid group had the largest number of final culture pathogens. This group also showed the largest number of cases of persistence of *Staphylococcus aureus*. The gentamicin treatment group, by contrast, showed the fewest (4 of 17, with an additional case showing pseudomonas).

The "bottom line" summarizes the bacteriological outcome of the study with respect to organisms generally assumed to be skin pathogens. At the end of treatment, 21 of 68 cultures remained pathogenic. Thus, the data indicate the relative efficacy, from a bacteriological point of view, of the three modalities.

Table VIII presents the totals of the physicians final evaluations of the results of treatment.

The data favor combination antibiotic/steroid therapy in the treatment of impetiginized atopic dermatitis over treatment with plain steroid ($p < 0.13$) and over plain antibiotic ($p < 0.0001$).

DISCUSSION

In the judgment of many clinicians, topical antibiotics may be sensitizing and do not necessarily enhance the effectiveness of corticoids. Others believe, equally firmly, that treatment with corticoids alone is potentially dangerous in that they may alter the body's natural resistance, mask the clinical manifestations of infection, and allow overgrowth of pathogens.

A recent *in vivo* and *in vitro* study by Raab (15, 16) reports some antibiotic/corticoid combinations more effective than their individual components in topical therapy of infected dermatoses. The antibacterial activity of gentamicin when combined with betamethasone valerate remained unimpaired and was superior to the other preparations studied. A study of these same agents by Kligman (17), employing quantitative

Table VIII. Summary of Physicians' Final Evaluations of Treatment
(% of Treatment Group)

	Excellent	Good	Fair	Poor
BV/G	18 (72%)	6 (20%)	2 (8%)	0 (0%)
BV	15 (56%)	5 (18%)	4 (15%)	3 (11%)[a]
G	8 (80%)	1 (4%)	7 (26%)	11 (41%)

[a]Includes one patient judged to have experienced an exacerbation.

bacterial counts, indicated a high degree of effectiveness and concluded with interesting epidemiologic implications. There have been other studies reported (18–21) which favor this combination, but none of the studies has been well controlled.

SUMMARY AND CONCLUSIONS

This paper reports the results of a double-blind controlled study of the treatment of impetiginized atopic dermatoses with a corticoid/ antibiotic combination cream, betamethasone valerate with gentamicin, evaluated against each of its active agents.

Both clinically and bacteriologically, the results favor the use of the combination cream. The data are not statistically significant at every point, but should not, in our opinion, be dismissed on that account. It may very well be that a larger study, involving perhaps 200 cases, would demonstrate the statistical significance—hence, the therapeutic validity— of the combination modality of treatment.

REFERENCES

1. H. Blank, Personal Communication, (1968).
2. C.M. Davis, *et al.*, The value of Neomycin in a Neomycin–steroid cream, *JAMA*. 203, 136–137 (1968).
3. W.G. Larsen, Topical Neomycin, *Arch. Derm.* 97, 202 (1968).
4. R.G. Carney, Topical use of antibiotics, *JAMA* 186, 646–648 (1963).
5. N.B. Esterly and M. Markowitz, The treatment of pyoderma in children, *JAMA* 212, 1667–1670 (1970).
6. W.E. Herrell, Editorial, *Clin. Med.* 19–20 (1968).

7. M.B. Sulzberger, Combined drugs important in skin disease treatment, *Skin and Allergy News*, 2 (1972).

8. C.L. Carpenter *et al.*, Combined anti-infective topical therapy in common dermatoses (Scientific Exhibit), *Amer. Acad. Family Physicians* (1972).

9. A. Kligman, In praise of what's old, *Derm. News* 7 (1973).

10. M.K. Polano, *et al.*, Analysis of results obtained in the treatment of atopic dermatitis with corticosteroid and Neomycin ointments, *Derm.* 120, 191–199 (1960).

11. R.R. Marples, A. Rebora, A.M. Kligman, Topical steroid–antibiotic combinations, *Arch. Derm.* 108, 237–240 (1973).

12. G. Wachs, R. Clark, and J. Hallet, Are topical steroid-related superinfections a myth? *Cutis* 10, 33 (1973).

13. K.M. Lloyd, Letter to the Editor. *Arch. Derm.* 109, 410 (1974).

14. J.J. Leyden, R.R. Marples, and A.M. Kligman, *Staphlococcus aureus* in the lesions of atopic dermatitis. *Brit. J. Derm.* 90, 525 (1974).

15. W. Raab, The interaction of corticosteroids and antimicrobial agents used in topical therapy, *Brit. J. Derm.* 84, 582–589 (1971).

16. W. Raab and Windisch: Corticosteroids versus antibiotics, *Derm.* 145, 400–402 (1973).

17. A. Kligman, Personal Communication (1971).

18. Y. Nakai, Increase in bacterial population of skin surface by ODT and the effect of addition of antibiotics to topical preparations, *Acta. Derm. (Kyoto)* 64, 25–34 (1969).

19. L. Bruni, Association of betamethasone valerate and gentamicin sulfate in the treatment of inflammatory dermatoses, *Min. Derm. (Italian Trans.)* 43, 89–96 (1968).

20. C.B. Sosa, Betamethasone valerate and gentamicin sulfate combination in the treament of some dermatoses, *Med. Rev. Mex. (Span.)* 998, 501–502 (1966).

21. M. Tonkin, *et al.*, Percutaneous absorption of a corticosteriod in combination with an antibiotic, *South African Med. J.* 1071–72 (1966).

22. J.J. Harris, A national double-blind clinical trial of a new corticosteroid lotion: A 12 investigator analysis, *Curr. Ther. Res.* 14, 638–644 (1972).

23. D.I. Williams, *et al.*, Betamethasone 17-valerate: a new corticosteroid, *The Lancet* I, 1174–79 (1964).

24. R.S. Higdon, *et al.*, Betamethasone valerate versus fluocinolone acetonide in cream base: clinical comparison by two separate institutions, *Cutis* 7, 563–566 (1971).

25. S.L. Fox, Aspects in diagnosis and management of external infections of the eye: Experiences with a new antibiotic, gentamicin, *South. Med. J.* 63, 1047–52 (1970).

26. S. Olansky, Topical therapy of pyodermas due to resistant bacterial strains. *Cutis* 2, 674–474 (1966).

Recent Advances in Dermatopharmacology

9

The Case for Steroid-Antibiotic Combinations

JAMES J. LEYDEN
ALBERT M. KLIGMAN

Topical steroid–antibiotic preparations are currently laboring under severe criticisms. Antagonists argue that rigorous scientific proof that combinations are superior to individual components has not been supplied. They decry "heedless exposure" to antibiotics citing the hazards of inducing resistant strains of pathogens and, in the case of neomycin, the risk of contact allergy. Despit these attacks, generalists and dermatologists prescribe such preparations widely. To some this represents an unwarranted "shotgun" approach, an unacceptable deviation from the goal of specific therapies for specific diagnoses.

The literature contains conflicting reports regarding the effectiveness of steroid–antibiotic combinations. For example, Lloyd did a parallel study of 45 cases of various impetiginized (infected) dermatoses; the healing rate was the same whether fluocinolone acetonide was used alone or in combination with 0.5% neomycin (1). However, he failed to recover a pathogen in fully a quarter of the cases, highlighting the unreliability of assessing secondary infection by inspection alone. It is worth noting that *Staphylococcus aureus* was completely eliminated in 47% of cases in 4 weeks with the combination while only 15% of those treated with the steroid alone became negative. A serious flaw in Lloyds methodology, evident in any other studies of this kind, is the failure to determine the quantity of organisms before and after treatment. Without quantitative cultures, cases which do not become entirely free of S. aureus are scored as antibiotic failures. This all-or-none type of analysis eliminates instances in which very significant reductions have been achieved. For example, a patient with a pretreatment count of millions of S. aureus per square centimeter falling to 1000/cm² after therapy would fall in the ineffective column despite a decrease of at least three orders of magnitude. Another factor which results in loss of discriminating power is inappropriate timing of observations. For example, combinations are most likely to effect clinically significant changes in the first 5 to 7 days. Lloyds clinical assessment was after 2 weeks.

Another controlled study which is a favorite among those who see no worth in combinations is that of Davis et al. (2). These workers failed to find a difference between 0.1 dexamethasone alone and in combination with .05%. Once again the diagnosis of an "infected" dermatoses was inaccurate. No pathogen could be demonstrated in a quarter of the cases. Again the quantity of virulent organisms was not determined before and after treatment. Leaving the failings aside, the design of the study precluded the possibility of showing a difference. The test agents were applied to opposite sites of the patient (symmetrical paired comparison method). Marples and Kligman have demonstrated that with potent antibiotics such as neomycin or chloranphenicol enough translocation occurs to produce degerming of distant untreated sites (3). The application of the antibiotic to a few square inches of skin on one arm will significantly suppress the microflora on the opposite side of the body. The surface concentration of neomycin that will inhibit multiplication of bacteria is only 4 μg/sq. cm (4). Therefore, in the study of Davis et al., twice daily application of 1% neomycin to one side was equivalent to treating both sides with the antibiotic. We have in fact repeatedly verified the translocation effect in atopic dermatitis lesions densely colonized with S. aureus. One other study, less well controlled than the above, also concluded that adding an antibiotic to the steroid did not enhance efficacy (5).

Other investigators believe they have demonstrated superiority for combinations, although the same methodologic criticisms apply. In impetiginized atopic dermatitis Polano and DeVries found that patients treated with a steroid–antibiotic combination achieved signficantly greater therapeutic effects than those on the steroid alone (6). Clark treated 40 cases of impetiginized dermatoses for 8 days with either fluocinolone acetonide or fluocinolone acetonide with neomycin. The combination was clinically superior; 15 of 20 patients treated with the combination achieved excellent results (more than 75% improved) compared to only 9 of 20 treated with the steroid alone (7).

Marples et al. utilized experimental human infections with *S. aureus* and *C. albicans* in order to assess the value of adding antibiotics to corticosteroids (8). Localized infections were induced permitting clinical and quantitative bacteriological assessment of efficacy with each component in comparison to the complete formulation. In this model the steroid–antibiotic combination proved to be superior to the steroid alone. Not only was inflammation moderated more quickly, but, as expected, the pathogens were rapidly suppressed or eliminated.

For whatever it is worth, one can cite evidence from the marketplace. Clinicians have overwhelmingly endorsed steroid–antibiotic combinations.

Our objective in this report is two-fold: (1) to give an account of the problems which underlie the current debate regarding steroid–antibiotic combinations, and (2) to demonstrate that in atopic dermatitis, a model disease for this purpose, the presence of an antibiotic adds to the clinical and bacteriological effectiveness of the steroid.

It is essential that the problem be explicitly stated. For the treatment of primary pyodermas (bullous impetigo, folliculitis, ecthyma, etc.) no one argues that the addition of a steroid will add anything to the efficacy of the antibiotic; the latter alone is curative. The debate revolves around the issue of whether an antibiotic should be added to a steroid in the treatment of chronic dermatoses such as atopic dermatitis; seborrheic dermatitis, etc.

The distinction between primary and secondary pyodermas is a crucial one to the issue at hand. In the former, a pathogen invades skin which was previously normal. *Staphylococcus aureus* and *Streptocooccus pyogenes* cause virtually all primary pyodermas. The case is entirely different in the case of secondary pyodermas. Here the basic condition is a chronic inflammatory process which becomes secondarily infected. It is well established by now that *S. aureus* commonly colonizes chronically inflamed skin while betahemolytic streptococci are rarely encountered (9–12).

One must come to grips with a vexing problem that has confounded many workers. What are the criteria for diagnosing secondary infection in dermatoses? For some, the mere isolation of *S. aureus* is evidence of "infection." This seems an oversimplification to us, for nearly every

Table I. Topical Vs. Oral Antibiotic Treatment of Atopic Dermatitis

Treatment	Subjects	Pretreatment S. aureus/cm^2		Posttreatment S. aureus/cm^2		
1% Neomycin,	13	Mean	360,000	Mean	388	(7)
BID		(Range	232 - 8,421,000)		0	(6)
Erythromycin	10	Mean	1,7000,000	Mean	1890	(7)
250 mg q.i.d.		(Range	1,000 - 22,000,000)		0	(3)

persistent inflammatory eruption will contain some *S. aureus*. The really important question for clinicians is whether or not the presence of *S. aureus* has any significance. When is the lesion infected and when are they merely colonized? This involves a dimension of quantification. We determined the density of *S. aureus* in a variety of chronic dermatoses. The numbers varied considerably in different disorders (11). In atopic dermatitis *S. aureus* was present in high numbers in virtually every case while in psoriasis the organism could be recovered in only about half the cases, usually in comparatively low numbers.

We have proposed that a lesion can be said to be infected when the burden of *S. aureus is* great enough to add to morbidity in some demonstrable way, that is to say, when the underlying disease is worsened. This is best illustrated by data from an actual study (13). We compared twice daily application of 1% neomycin cream to 250 mg. of erythromycin given orally, q.i.d., in suppressing *S. aureus* in atopic dermatitis. *Staphylococcus aureus* was sharply suppressed by both treatments, more by topical neomycin. The most important finding in this study was that an appreciable degree of clinical improvement occurred only in those patients whose lesions harbored more than 10 *S. aureus* per cm.^{2} before treatment (13). It was not expected that the lesions would clear and indeed this never happened; the underlying process persisted. We consider that *S. aureus* is likely to be aggravating the primary disease when the density reaches 1×10^6/cm^2 or higher. Such numbers are by no means unusual in exudative chronic dermatoses. It cannot be too strongly emphasized that the traditional criteria for judging infection are unreliable. Suppuration, tenderness, adenopathy, and fever are usually absent. By the time impetiginization occurs, that is crusting and pus, the *S. aureus* count has reached tens of millions per sq cm. The educated observer, however, can often sense early

Table II. Comparison of Steroid and Antibiotic
Applied Under Occlusion to Atopic Dermatitis

Treatment	Pretreatment[a] $S.\ aureus/cm^2$	72 Hours occlusion	
		$S.\ aureus/cm^2$	Clinical
1% Neomycin	1,200,000 (700,000 - 4,000,000)	12,600	25% Improvement
0.025% Synalar	1,600,000 (1,200,000 - 3,200,000)	13,400,000	25-50% Worse
Control	1,400,000 (800,000 - 3,400,000)	20,000,000	50-75% Worse

[a]Geometric means.

impetiginization by close clinical inspection. Another way of demonstrating that high levels of S. aureus can aggravate the underlying lesions is to arrange for its increase. This can be accomplished by simple occlusion as the following study illustrates. Three 5 cm squares were marked out on skin afflicted with atopic dermatitis. Each square received either 0.1 mil of 0.025% of fluocinolone acetonide cream (Synalar,® Syntex), 0.1 ml of 0.25% fluocinolone acetonide plus 0.5% neomycin sulfate (Neo-Synlar®, Syntex), or 0.1 ml of USP vanishing cream (control). The sites were covered with impermeable polyethylene films and then occlusively taped to the skin. The dressings were left in place for 72 hours. Before and afterwards the sites were assessed clinically and bacteriologically. (Table II) The control sites (*S. aureus,* $10 \times 10^6/cm^2$) showed a marked aggravation of the dermatitis; the lesion was redder, more edematous, and exudative. This worsening was partially blocked by steroid alone despite vast increase in S. aureus. The antiinflammatory activity of the steroid accounts for this moderating effect. These results contrast with the usual benefit seen with repeated applications of topical steroid under occlusive dressings. With repeated application (as opposed to one application for 72 hours) clinical improvement routinely occurs. By contrast, with neomycin, not only was there no intensification but an unmistakeable clinical improvement occurred.

We think it important to describe in detail two double-blind studies which we conducted to test the hypothesis that steroid–antibiotic combinations are superior to the individual components. The patients, mainly children, had typical but rather severe atopic dermatitis; they were recruited from the dermatology clinic at the Hospital of the University of Pennsylvania. None were using antibacterial soaps or had received antibiotic therapy for the previous month.

In the first study, 34 patients were randomly assigned to either a 0.025% fluocinolone acetonide cream (Synalar®, Syntex) or the same cream with 0.5% neomycin sulfate (Neo-Synalar®, Syntex). The cream was applied twice daily for 1 week. In the second study, a combination of polymyxin B, neomycin sulfate, gramididin cream (Neosporin®, Burroughs–Wellcome) was compared to the same cream with .05% hydrocortisone (Cortisporin®, Burroughs–Wellcome). The latter study differed from the first study in that the test agents were applied to opposite sides and not to different patients. The bilateral paired comparison method was an acceptable design in the second study because both sides received the antibiotics and translocation effects are not noticeable with steroids, especially low-potency ones, like hydrocortisone.

Clinical improvement was evaluated for the following parameters: (1) pruritus; (2) erythema; (3) lichenification; (4) oozing and crusting; (5) scaling.

The scoring system was: $0 =$ none; $1 =$ mild; $2 =$ moderate; $3 =$ severe. A 75% or greater reduction in grades was recorded as excellent, 50 to 75% reduction as good; 25 to 50% as fair; 0 to 25% as poor.

Quantitative cultures were obtained by the detergent scrub technique. In brief this method employs two 1-minute scrubbings with Triton-X-100 (Rohm and Haas Co., Phila.) in a 3.8 sq cm. area of skin delineated by a sterile cup (14). Samples were pooled, serially diluted, and drop plated on appropriate media.

RESULTS

Study I (Synalar Vs. Neo-Synalar)

Bacteriology

Staphylococcus aureus was the dominant organism and constituted more than 90% of the total flora in both groups having mean pretreatment *S. aureus* counts of $200,000/cm^2$ (Synalar) and $420,000/cm^2$ (Neo-Synalar). After one week of the steroid alone the count was reduced to $65,000/cm^2$ (not significant) while the combination reduced the count to $350/cm^2$ (highly significant). With the combination, *S. aureus* was completely eradicated in 12 of 15 subjects; by contrast 13 of 21 patients treated with the steroid alone still supported *S. aureus* at a mean density of $65,000/cm^2$.

Table III. Steroid-Antibiotic Combinations in Atopic Dermatitis Bacteriology Results (geometric mean counts per sq cm)

Agent	N	Pretherapy		Posttherapy		Significance[a]
		Total Aerobic Flora	S. aureus	Total Aerobic Flora	S. aureus	
Synalar	21	253,000	200,000	73,700	65,000 ⎫	p < 0.01
Neo-Synalar	15	426,000	420,000	688	350 ⎬	
Cortisporin	25	4,100,000	4,000,000	8,500	1,200 ⎫	N.S.
Neosporin	25	2,010,000	1,900,000	500	80 ⎬	

Clinical response

Response	Synalar (%)	Neo-Synalar (%)	Neosporin (%)	Cortisporin (%)
Excellent	30	70	0	12
Good	40	20	12	64
Fair	30	10	68	24
No change	–	–	20	–

[a]Significance was assessed by the Wilcoxin summed rank test.

Clinical Response

Neo-Synalar produced excellent results in 70% of subjects compared to 30% of those treated with Synalar alone. Each subject who achieved excellent results with the combination harbored at least 1,000,000/cm² of S. aureus; those achieving excellent results with the steroid alone initially supported low numbers of S. aureus (a mean of 150,000 per sq cm). Good results (50 to 75% improvement) were attained by 40% of those treated with fluocinolone alone.

Study II (Cortisporin Vs. Neosporin)

Bacteriology

Again, S. aureus was the dominant organism and constituted more than 95% of the total flora, the mean pre-treatment counts being 4,000,-000/cm² (Cortisporin) and 1,900,000/cm² (Neosporin). After 1 week of therapy, the mean aerobic density for Cortisporin was 8,500/cm² for Neosporin and 500 for Cortisporin. Both treatments produced a highly significant reduction in S. aureus and there was no significant difference between the two agents.

Clinical Response

Cortisporin produced excellent results in 12%, good in 64%, and fair in 24%. With Neosporin no subject had an excellent result, while 12% had good results, and 68% fair.

Comment

In both studies, the combination was unequivically superior in respect to clinical improvement. The greater clinical efficacy of the fluocinolone combination doubtless reflects the greater anti-inflammatory potency of the fluorinated steroid. It cannot be denied that the fluorinated steroid alone had appreciable efficacy, producing an excellent result in about a third of the subjects. These were usually patients with comparatively low numbers of S. aureus. It must be noted however that S. aureus was not suppressed to a significant degree by the steroid alone, though indeed the trend was consistently downwards. Moderation of the dermatitis makes the habitat less suitable for S. aureus. Both steroid–antibiotic combinations virtually eliminated S. aureus in the great majority of patients. A mixture of antibiotic with a weak steroid, hydrocortisone (Cortisporin), strongly suppressed S. aureus, but clinical improvement was clearly less impressive than with fluorinated steroid. With the hydrocortisone combination, the best clinical results were attained in patients with very high S. *aureus* densities.

An instructive contrast is revealed in these two studies. When the S. *aureus* counts are low, a potent steroid is therapeutically equivalent to the steroid–antibiotic combination; an excellent result can be obtained with the steroid alone when there is no true secondary infection, i.e. the lesions are colonized by S. *aureus* but the density is not sufficient to aggravate the underlying process. On the other hand, when the steroid in a combination is a low potency one (hydrocortisone), excellent results are most often obtained when secondary infection exists ($>1 \times 10^6/cm^2$). It cannot be too strongly emphasized that barring gross impetiginization there is no way to estimate the density of S. *aureus* by clinical evaluation.

These studies demonstrated that in secondarily infected atopic dermatitis, steroid–antibiotic combinations produced superior clinical and bacteriological results in 1-week's time to either the steroid or antibiotic alone. Wachs has recently conducted a multicentered, double-blind study comparing bethamethasone valerate alone, gentamycin alone, and the combination in impetiginized atopic and contact dermatitis (15). Although S. *aureus* densities were not determined it was concluded that the combination was superior both by microbiological and clinical criteria. In atopic dermatitis, their results paralleled ours. After 1 week of therapy, the combination produced excellent (more than 75% clearing) clinical results in 73% and good results in 20%, compared to our findings of 70% and 20% with Neo-Synalar and Synalar. They found gentamycin alone produced good to excellent results in 33% of their cases of "impetiginized" atopic eczema compared to our findings of 12% with Neosporin. Presumably nearly all these cases were secondarily infected as denoted by the clinical findings of impetiginization, whereas some of our subjects had comparatively low counts and would therefore not benefit from antibiotics alone.

Our studies support the concept that a dermatitis is secondarily infected when the level of S. *aureus* is in excess of 10^6 organisims/cm.^{2} At this density S. *aureus* is aggravating the underlying inflammatory process. When the S. *aureus* counts exceed $10^7/cm^2$ signs of frank infection may emerge. In the usual instance, the eye cannot identify the early infection because the classic signs are masked by the underlying inflammatory disease. Still with increasing experience one is able to sense, by the intensity of the dermatitis, whether or not the S. *aureus* level is low or high.

Antibiotics alone are helpful in frankly infected cases while antibiotic–steroid combinations are characteristically capable of producing moderate to marked clearing depending on the potency of the steroid. Fluorinated steroids alone are unquestionably helpful in nearly all cases, especially when secondary infection is absent.

Quantitative bacteriology is not available to the practitioner; he must act on the spot and rely on experience in deciding whether an antibiotic will be helpful. We have been impressed that clinicians very commonly initiate treatment of steroid-sensitive disorders with a course of antibiotics. These diseases include atopic dermatitis, numular eczema, chronic contact dermatitis, external otitis, diaper dermatitis,, intertrigo, etc. The tradition of empiricism in medicine gains strength from such practices which were not based on perceiving that frank infection exists, but are based instead on the beneficial changes wrought by the therapy. Our observations on inapparant infection provide a rationalization for such long standing clinical practices. We hasten to make it clear that we do not advocate combinations for all chronic dermatoses. In a dry dermatoses such as psoriasis little is to be gained by adding an antibiotic to the steroid. The reason for this is that only about half the cases carry *S. aureus* and then usually in low or moderate numbers. In intertriginous areas, diaper dermatitis, for example, one also has to contend with yeasts such as *C. albicans* and occasionally gram negatives. Given the variety of diseases and the complexity of the microflora, it is scarcely surprising that practitioners, including skin specialists, often resort to multiaction medicaments. Steroid–antibiotic combinations provide some security in the all too frequent predicament of undiagnosable dermatoses in which a melange of causative factors are operating. We advocate combination therapy for those conditions in which the microbial components cannot be precisely identified by clinical study alone. For certain of these we endorse combinations which contain several types of antibiotics to provide broad-spectrum coverage against gram positives, gram negative, and yeasts. Typical examples would be diaper rash, otitis externa, and intertriginous eruptions.

The question must be raised whether harm can result from injudicious use of steroid–antibiotic combinations. The main objections are those of contact allergy and the development of resistant organisms.

What amounts to a holy furor has been raised concerning the allergenicity of neomycin. The key question relates to the prevalence of contact allergic dermatitis to this agent. Most of the data implicating neomycin as a "leading" sensitizer stem from clinics where patients with chronic, often unclassifiable, inflammatory dermatoses are subjected to batteries of patch tests. In this highly selected population, neomycin sensitivity is fairly frequent. The North American Contact Dermatitis group, for example, found contact allergic dermatitis (16). In this highly selected group, neomycin ranked in the top 10 of the most frequently encountered sensitizers. The European group diagnoses neomycin allergy in 3.7% of 4,825 patients with chronic undiagnosed dermatoses and ranked neomycin among the top 20 contact allergens (17).

The frequency of reactions in patients attending dermatology clinics has created the impression that neomycin is a potent sensitizer. The widespread use of neomycin in topical antibiotics and at one time in deodorants make it very unlikely that sensitization develops at an unacceptably high rate. If this were so, neomycin would by now have followed the path of penicillin and been driven off the market. The majority of contact allergies follow prolonged application to chronically inflammed skin. Susceptibility appears to be particularly great in patients with stasis dermatitis and stasis ulcers (18). When that group is excluded, the prevalence of neomycin allergy falls drastically. The message is that steroid–antibiotic combinations containing neomycin should not be used indefinitely, particularly on chronic eruptions of the lower legs. Brief or intermittent use does not appear to carry a high risk of sensitization.

Another frequently raised objection is that widespread use of topical neomycin leads to resistant strains, particularly S. aureus. It is assertd that these same strains are also resistant to penicillin and that such strains are commonly involved in septicemias (19). Existing reports, however, do not support such statements. There is convincing evidence that widespread use of topical neomycin in a closed population such as a hospital ward can lead to the emergence of neomycin resistant strains; these can be involved in wound infections (20,21). Only one report described resistant strains in 32 of 442 strains of S. aureus isolated from pyodermas in an outpatient population (22). Actually, the latter was virtually a closed community with high contact between the members. It turns out, in fact, that resistant strains are characteristically Group III strains and are rarely the more virulent 70/71, 80/81 varieties. These Group III strains have been on rare occasions responsible for pneumonia and enterocoloitis but not septicemias. Cohen et al., reported that the S. aureus was accompanied by a disappearance of S. aureus septicemia (23).

There is no evidence linking the use of neomycin in outpatients to any serious hazard. On the other hand, there is considerable evidence that the failure to eliminate S. aureus from chronically inflamed skin can occasionally lead to public health disasters. Dermatitic skin, as we and others have shown, is characteristically colonized by S. *aureus*. These are dispersed into the environment on desquamating scales leading to a significant contamination of the environment with potential pathogens. The usual strains of S. *aureus* are relatively nonvirulent but on occasion the strain can cause severe wound infections and even deaths (24,25). One anesthetist in England, for example, dispersed a virulent S. *aureus* from his psoriasis; four patients died of infections with the same organism. We have observed an epidemic of 8 post-operative, severe wound infections due to S. *aureus*. The source was traced to the hand eczema of the ward resident. While his eruption did not appear "clinically infected," more than 10^6 S. *aureus* per sq cm were repeatedly recovered. Antibiotiograms and phage typing confirmed the identity of his S. *aureus* and that recovered from the wounds.

Both clinical observations and the controlled studies reported here indicate that steroid–antibiotic combinations offer a scientifically sound therapeutic approach to the management of secondarily infected derma-toses. We would suggest the following guidelines for such therapy; (1) If feasible, cultures are advisable before therapy. In nonresponsive cases extraordinary efforts may be justified to determine the kinds and numbers of organisms; (2) steroid–antibiotic combinations are best used early in management (first week or two). Once S. *aureus* is eliminated or reduced to a harmless level, steroids alone will suffice; (3) long term use of topical antibiotics should be avoided particularly for stasis der-matitis and stasis ulcers; (4) the selection of which combination to use depends on the area involved and the likely complicating organisms. In the case of secondarily infected dermatoses of the glaborous skin, S. *aureus* is by far the most common organism and a neomycin–steroid combination would be sufficient. In intertriginous lesions one also has to contend with C. *albicans* and gram negatives, therefore broad-spec-trum combinations are indicated.

REFERENCES

1. K.M. Lloyd, The value of neomycin in topical corticosteroid prepara-tions. *South Med. J.* 62, 94–96 (1964).
2. C.M. Davis, D.D. Fulghum, D. Taplin, The value of neomycin in a neomycin–steroid cream. *JAMA* 202, 298–300 (1968).
3. R.R. Marples and A.M. Kligman, Limitation of paired comparisons of topical drugs. *Brit. J. Derm.* 88, 61–67 (1973).

4. R.R. Marples and A.M. Kligman, Methods for evaluating topical anti-bacterial agents on human skin. *Antimicrobial Agents and Chemoth.* 5, 323–329 (1974).

5. S. Friedlaender and A.S. Friedlaender, Topical use of hydrocortisone and hydrocortisone–neomycin ointments in allergic dermatoses. *J. Allergy* 25, 417–428 (1954).

6. M.K. Polano and H.R. DeVries, Analysis of the results obtained in the treatment of atopic dermatitis with corticosteroid- and neomycin-containing ointments. *Dermatologica* 120, 191–199 (1960).

7. R.F. Clark, The case for corticosteroid–antibiotic combinations. *Cutis* 14, 737–741 (1974).

8. R.R. Marples, A. Reborah, and A.M. Kligman, Topical steroid–antibiotic combinations. *Arch. Derm.* 108, 237–240 (1973).

9. S. Selwyn and D. Chalmers, Dispersal of bacteria from skin lesions: A hospital hazard. *Brit. J. Derm.* 77, 349–354 (1965).

10. W.C. Noble, The dispersal of staphylococci in hospital wards. *J. Clin. Path.* 15, 552 (1962).

11. J.J. Leyden, Antibiotic usage in dermatological practice. *Inter. J. Derm.* 13, 342–352 (1974).

12. S. Selwyn, Bacterial infections in a skin department. *Brit. J. Derm.* 75, 26 (1963).

13. J.J. Leyden and R.R. Marples, *S. aureus* in the lesions of atopic dermatitis. Brit. J. Derm. 90, 552–530 (1974).

14. P. Williamson and A.M. Kligman, A new method for the quantitative investigation of cutaneous bacteria. *J. Invest. Dermatol.* 45, 498 (1965).

15. G.N. Wachs and H. I. Maibach, A nationwide double-blind analysis of an antibiotic steroid combination in Impetiginized Dermatoses. *Brit. J. Derm.*, (1976), in press.

16. North American Contact Dermatitis Research Group, Epidemiology of contact dermatitis in North America: 1972. *Arch. Derm.* 108, 537–540 (1973).

17. S. Ferget, et al., Epidemiology of contact dermatitis. *Trans. St. John's Hospital Dermatol. Soc.* 55, 17–35 (1969).

18. K. Wereide, Neomycin sensitivity in atopic dermatitis and eczematous conditions. *Acta Dermatotoven* 50, 114–116 (1970).

19. F.J. Storrs, Treatment of nonbullous impetigo. *Cutis* 16: 886–892 (1975).

20. V.G. Alder, W.A. Billespie, Influence of neomycin sprays on the spread of resistant staphylococci. *Lancet* 2, 1062–1063 (1962).

21. E.J. Lowbry, J.R. Babb and V.I. Brown, et al., Neomycin resistant *Staphylococcus aureus* in a burn unit. *J. Hyg. Comb.* 62, 221–228 (1964).

22. B.F. Anthony, G.S. Griehink and P.G. Quie, Neomycin resistant staphylococci in a rural outpatient population. *Amer. J. Dis. Child* 113, 664–672 (1967).

23. L.S. Cohen, F.R. Feketry and L.E. Clough, Studies on the epidemiology

of staphyloccal infection. The changing ecology of hospital staphylococci. *N.E.J. Med.* 266, 367–374 (1962).

24. R.W. Payne, Severe outbreak of surgical sepsis due to *Staphylococcus aureus* of unusual type and origin. *Brit. Med. J.* 4, 17 (1967).

25. G.A. Ayliffe and B.J. Collins, Wound infections from a disperser of an unusual strain of *Staphylococcus aureus. J. Clin. Path.* 10, 195 (1967).

10

Evaluation of New Potent Steroids

RICHARD B. STOUGHTON

Try to imagine, if you can, practicing dermatology without gluco-corticosteroids. What will you give the patient with hand eczema? What will you give to the patient with flexural atopic dermatitis? What will you give for widespread neurodermatitis, localized areas of psoriasis, seborrheic dermatitis, pruritic dermatoses? It is a fact that half the prescriptions written by dermatologists are for glucocorticosteroids, mostly, of course, topical glucocorticosteroids. The international market for topical glucocorticoids is close to a half billion dollars per year.

The original trials of topical steroids were with cortisone acetate, which was totally ineffective and almost doomed the entire future of topical steroid therapy (1). However, curiosity prevailed and hydro-cortisone was then tried with fairly dramatic results (2,3). Since that time, as we all know, there have been many new glucocorticosteroids and various formulations that have been introduced. There is no question that there is an enormously wide range in the spectrum of activity of these preparations. This paper attempts to delineate this spectrum and the bases for judgments on the relative activities of the myriad of preparations available to the practicing physician.

DEVELOPMENTAL ASSAY TECHNIQUES

First, it must be stated that the many tests of potency which involve organ systems other than the skin are practically useless in predicting potency by topical application. It is a part of the unpleasant past and it will not be useful to review these consistent failures.

I do not attempt to cover all the topical assay techniques as there is not space and many are inadequate, unproved, and of historical interest only. However, there are a number of assays which do have direct relevance to predicting the potency of a glucocorticosteroid by topical application. They are as follows: (1) Vasoconstriction assay (Stoughton and McKenzie; 4,5); (2) Sholtz-Dumas assay (6); (3) Ultraviolet-light erthema suppression (7); (4) Croton oil assay (8); (5) Tetrahydrofurfuryl alcohol assay (9).

1. The vasoconstrictor assay is probably the most widely used tool to screen new steroids and formulations (10-15). The basic screening of different steroids is conducted on human volunteers with application of graded concentrations in ethanol to the forearms. The lowest concentration giving vasoconstriction in over 50% (ED50) of the subjects is taken as the endpoint. The steroids are applied under occlusion for 16–20 hours before reading. Because of the importance of the vehicle in controlling penetration of the incorporated steroid a modification of the assay is required. The formulation is applied (5–10 mg/3.6cm²) to the forearms and is proteced by an elevated guard which does not occlude but does protect the area. The reason for this modification is that occlusion will vastly enhance penetration and will obscure significant formulation differences that may exist. This assay is most practical because in clinical use the formulation is applied and there is no protection of the treated area. Thus, clothing, washing, friction, etc., may grossly interfere with effectiveness of a formulation. To account for this, another modification of the assay is employed in which the formulations are applied and no protective covering or occlusive wraps are used.

2. The Sholtz–Dumas assay employs the clinical lesion, usually psoriasis, to evaluate the steroid formulation. The formulation is applied to small areas of a psoriatic plaque and covered with occlusive wrap. Reapplication to the same area is employed over many days to see what happens to the psoriasis in the area of application. This is a valuable technique but has some problems, the main one being the use of occlusion, which tends to eliminate significant differences between the differ-

ent formulations and obscure important differences in formulations which will be apparent in clinical use where occlusion is not used.

3. Ultraviolet-light (UVL) erythema suppression was employed early in steroid development but without much success. The main reason for the lack of success was that the earlier steroids were too weak to detect by this technique. Further work with more potent topical steroids reveals that UVL erythema can be suppressed if applied within 4–8 hours of the UVL exposure and if the UVL erythema is not too intense (preferably less than 5 minimum erythema doses). The ranking of steroids and formulations with the UVL technique closely parallels that obtained with the standard vasoconstriction technique (16).

4. The croton oil assay has been used sporadically for many years (8). The results are at some variance with the other assays but the general trend is similar. The main problem is that it is much more difficult to conduct the assay as compared to the vasoconstriction technique.

5. The tetrahydrofurfuryl assay (9) was one of the original techniques and relied on the suppression of erythema induced by the tetrahydrofurfuryl when the steroid was dissolved in it and then applied under patches. It is also an occlusive technique. In general, the results of this assay parallel the results of the vasoconstriction assay.

Once the basic assay procedures have identified steroids and formulations of potential use it is essential to use clinical testing to verify the activity in a practical setting. These techniques are well known to everyone but a few words of comment, particularly caution, might be in order.

The double-blind paired-comparison technique is the most useful clinical assay, in my opinion. However, it can be useless if it is not done with understanding of the potential difficulties and pitfalls. You *must* have intelligent and cooperative patients who are highly motivated to take part in a research protocol. The casual use of standard teaching clinics and resident staff physicians is probably the worst setting for this type of study. The most effective method, in my experience, has been working with members of a chapter of the National Psoriasis Foundation. These people who suffer from psoriasis are extremely motivated to participate in drug evaluations, listen carefully to directions, and meticulously follow a protocol outlined for them.

Random assignments of one preparation per subject in the comparison of two preparations is a very poor way to differentiate clinical activities of formulations unless there is an enormous difference such as that between hydrocortisone 1% ointment and Lidex cream. More subtle differences will not appear from this type of clinical study short of many hundreds of cases. When you can distinguish subtle differences with only 30 patients in a well conducted double-blind paired-comparison study it seems folly to even consider the above, random assignment, method of study.

The crudest test of all is the judgment of clinicians in open use of the formulation without any controls. However, even though crude, it is invaluable in that it is the only testing method that will allow observations on thousands of patients. This is the test of the marketplace. It is quite interesting that this test (based on sales volume) quite accurately reflects the ranking of steroid formulations by the vasoconstrictor assay and double-blind paired-comparison assays.

With this as an introduction, it is time to discuss the more potent preparations that are now available as prescription drugs. Table 1 shows a ranking of glucocorticosteroid formulations that are now available for clinical use. This ranking is based on vasoconstrictor assays, double-blind studies, and general clinical observations. It includes information from the literature as well as some of our own personal observations. It should be emphasized that this ranking is a general guide and outline and not a rigid, unchallengeable edict. There are no major differences of the steroid formulations within each group but there are definite differences between the groups.

Also, Table 2 lists many of the steroid formulations that are available by generic and trade name and by concentration of the glucocorticosteroid.

The more potent a topical formulation is clinically, the more likely it is to induce undesirable side effects. In addition to the disturbances of the pituitary–adrenal axis, the stronger topical steroids are capable of inducing the following: (1) Senile type purpura; (2) rosacea-like eruption of face; (3) severe exacerbation of acne vulgaris; (4) epidermal and dermal atrophy; (5) striae; (6) glaucoma (reported but not proved); and (7) exacerbation of dermatophyte infections.

Recently, it has been shown that repeated applications of strong topical steroids can result in a diminishing biologic effect of the same preparation (17). This has been shown very clearly for the vasoconstrictor activity of triamcinolone acetonide and Lidex cream (17). This phenomenon, known to pharmacologists as tachyphylaxis, may also be operative in clinical disease. Further investigation of this property of strong steroids may help in setting up optimum regimens for the topical management of responsive dermatoses. Possibly related to this tachy-

Table I. Order of Potency[a]

I.	Halog cream 0.1% Lidex cream 0.05% Lidex ointment 0.05% Topsyn gel 0.05%
II.	Diprosone cream 0.05% Valisone ointment 0.1% Fluorobate gel (Benisone gel) 0.025% Aristocort cream 0.5% Valisone lotion 0.1%
III.	Synalar ointment 0.025% Cordran ointment 0.05% Kenalog ointment 0.1% Aristocort ointment 0.1% Synalar cream (HP) 0.2%
IV.	Kenalog cream 0.1% Synalar cream 0.025% Cordran cream 0.05% Kenalog lotion 0.025% Valisone cream 0.1%
V.	Locorten cream 0.03% Desonide cream 0.05%
VI.	Topicals with hydrocortisone, dexamethasone, flumethalone, prednisolone and methyl prednisolone

[a]Group I is most potent and potency descends with each group to Group VI which is least potent. There is no significant difference of agents within any given group.

phylaxis is the "rebound phenomenon" which has been widely observed in management of psoriasis by systemically administered glucocorticosteroids. "Rebound" from topical application of steroids for psoriasis has not really been discussed but has been observed by the author on a few but dramatic occasions. It is probably a more important factor than has been realized in the management of dermatoses with the more potent topical steroids.

Table II. Some Glucocorticoids for Topical Use

Generic name	Trade name

Betamethasone-17-benzoate	Benisone
	  gel (0.025)
	Flurobate
	  gel (0.025)

Betamethasone diproprionate	Diprosone cream (0.05)

Betamethasone-17-valerate	Valisone
	  cream (0.1)
	  ointment (0.1)
	  lotion (0.1)
	  aerosol

Desonide	Tridesilon cream (0.05)
Dexamethasone	Aeroseb-D aerosol
Flumethasone pivalate	Locorten cream (0.03)

Fluocinolone acetonide	Synalar
	  cream (0.025; 0.01)
	  ointment (0.025)
	  solution (0.01)
	  emollient cream (0.025)
	Synalor-HP
	  cream (0.2)
	Neo-Synalar (Neomycin)
	  cream (0.025)
	Fluonid
	  cream (0.025; 0.01)
	  ointment (0.025)
	  solution (0.01)

Fluocinolone acetonide acetate	Lidex
	  cream (0.05)
	  ointment (0.05)
	Topsyn
	  gel (0.05)

Fluorometholone	Oxylone cream (0.025)

Flurandrenolide	Cordran
	  cream (0.05; 0.025)
	  ointment (0.05; 0.025)
	  lotion (0.05)
	  tape (4 mcg/cm^2)

110

Generic name	Trade name
Halcinonide	Halog cream (0.1)
Hydrocortisone (Only a few representative formulations are given)	Cort-Dome cream (0.5; 1.0) lotion (0.5; 1.0) Lubricort cream (0.25; 0.5; 1.0) lotion (0.25; 0.5; 1.0)
Hydrocortisone acetate (Only a few representative formulations are given)	Cortef ointment (1.0; 2.5) Carmol HC (urea 10%) cream (1.0) Neo-Cortef (Neomycin) cream (1.0; 2.5)
Methylprednisolone acetate	Medrol Acetate Topical cream (0.25; 1.0)
Prednisolone	Meti-Derm cream (0.5) aerosol
Triamcinolone acetonide	Kenalog cream (0.1; 0.025) ointment (0.1; 0.025) lotion (0.1; 0.025) spray Orabase (0.1%) Kenalog S lotion (0.1) ⎧ Neomycin cream (0.1) ⎨ Gramicidin ointment (0.1) Mycolog (Nystatin; Neomycin; Gramicidin) ointment (0.1) cream (0.1) Aristocort cream (0.5; 1.0; 0.025) ointment (0.1) Aristoderm foam (0.1) NeoAristoderm (Neomycin) foam (0.1) Neo-Aristocort cream (0.1) ⎫ (Neomycin) ointment (0.1) ⎭

ACKNOWLEDGMENT

Supported by Research Grant No. AM 11649 from the National Institutes of Health.

REFERENCES

1. L. Goldman, R.G. Thompson and E.R. Trice, Cortisone acetate in skin disease. *Arch. Derm. Syph.* 65, 177–186 (1952).
2. M.B. Sulzberger and V.H. Witten, The effect of topically applied compound F in selected dermatoses. *J. Invest. Dermatol.* 19, 101–102 (1952).
3. M.B. Sulzberger and V.H. Witten, Hydrocortisone ointment in dermatological therapy. *Med. Clin. N. Amer.* 38, 321 (1954).
4. A.W. McKenzie, Percutaneous absorption of steroids. *Arch. Dermatol.* 86, 611–614 (1962).
5. A.W. McKenzie and R.B. Stoughton, Method for comparing percutaneous absorption of steroids. *Arch. Dermatol.* 86, 608–610 (1962).
6. J.R. Scholtz and K.J. Dumas, Standards for clinical evaluation of topical steroids. 13th International Congress of Dermatology. pp. 179–181. Springer-Verlag, New York, 1968.
7. A. Scott and F. Kalz, The effect of the topical application of corticotrophin, hydrocortisone and fluorocortisone on the process of cutaneous inflammation. *J. Invest. Dermatol.* 26, 361–378 (1956).
8. J.A. Witkowski and A.M. Kligman. A screening test for anti-inflammatory activity using human skin. *J. Invest. Dermatol.* 32, 481–483 (1959).
9. C.A. Schlagel, Comparative efficacy of topical anti-inflammatory corticosteroids. *J. Pharm. Sci.* 54, 335–354 (1965).
10. A.W. McKenzie and R.M. Atkinson, Topical activities of betamethasone esters in man. *Arch Dermatol.* 89, 741–746 (1964).
11. B.J. Poulsen, E. Young, V. Coqiulla, et al., Effect of topical vehicle composition on the in vitro release of fluocinolone acetonide and its acetate ester. *J. Pharm. Sci.* 57, 928–933 (1968).
12. R.B. Stoughton, Vasoconstrictor activity and percutaneous absorption of glucocorticosteroids. *Arch. Dermatol.* 99, 753–756 (1969).
13. R.B. Stoughton, (Personal observations).
14. R.B. Stoughton, Corticosteroids in psoriasis, in "Psoriasis, Proceedings of the International Symposium." (Eugene M. Farber, Alvin J. Cox, eds.) pp. 367–375. Stanford University Press, Stanford, 1971.
15. J. Ostrenga, J. Haleblian, B. Poulsen, et al., Vehicle design for a new topical steroid, fluocinonide. *J. Invest. Dermatol.* 56, 392–399 (1971).
16. R.B. Stoughton, (Personal observations).
17. A. du Vivier and R.B. Stoughton, Tachyphylaxis to the action of topically applied corticosteroids. *Arch. Dermatol.* 111, 581–583 (1975).

11

Relation of Vehicle to Corticosteroid Potency

MATTHEW A. AUGUSTINE

The effect of the vehicle on the efficacy of topically active steroids has only recently been recognized as an important factor in formulation design studies. As has been reported by Poulsen (1), Katz and Poulsen (2), and Scheuplein and Blank (3), among others, knowledge of the physicochemical relationships between drug-vehicle and skin is necessary in order to formulate effective therapeutic products.

This study concerns itself with the evaluation of four chemically related 21-chloro-substituted steroids, originally found to be active when screened in the human vasoconstrictor and stripped skin assays, and the importance of their physicochemical properties which were considered in their evaluation as potential products for use in dermatology. The data presented in this study has appeared, in part, elsewhere (4,5). The four test steroids together with betamethasone-17-valerate are shown in Figure 1. Both SQ15,361 and SQ18,566, which are generically known as halcinonide, contain a flourine atom in the 9-α position, whereas SQ20,589 and SQ20,811 are their respective desfluoro analogs. Both SQ15,361 and SQ20,589 contain double bonds at the one and four position in the A ring, while the remaining two steroids have a single

9 α-FLUORO-11 β,17 α, 21-TRIHYDROXY-16 β-METHYLPREGNA-
1,4-DIENE-3,20-DIONE 17-VALERATE (BETAMETHASONE VALERATE)

9 α-FLUORO-21-CHLORO-11 β, 16 α, 17 α-TRIHYDROXYPREGNA-
1,4-DIENE 3,20-DIONE, 16,17-ACETONIDE. (SQ 15,361)

9 α-FLUORO-21-CHLORO-11 β,16 α,17 α-TRIHYDROXYPREGN-4-
ENE-3,20-DIONE, 16,17-ACETONIDE. (SQ 18,566)

1 Chemical structures of betamethasone valerate and candidate topical steroids.

21-CHLORO-11 β, 16 α, 17 α TRIHYDROXYPREGNA-1,4-DIENE
3,20-DIONE, 16,17-ACETONIDE. (SQ 20,589)

21 CHLORO 11 β, 16 α, 17 α TRIHYDROXYPREGN 4 ENE
3,20 DIONE, 16,17 ACETONIDE. (SQ 20,811)

114

Table I. Solubility Profile of Candidate Steroids as a
Function of Propylene Glycol Concentration.[1]

Compound	Percent Propylene Glycol (w/w)			
	30	40	60	100
SQ 15,361	0.0003	0.0006	0.0015	0.021
SQ 18,566	0.0017	0.0033	0.015	0.270
SQ 20,589	0.0002	0.0004	0.0022	0.027
SQ 20,811	0.002	0.0028	0.04	0.125

[1]Room temperature

double bond in the 4 position. Betamethasone-17-valerate was used as the reference compound in most of the biological studies.

The room temperature solubilities of these test steroids as a function of the concentration of propylene glycol in water were determined and are shown in Table I. A propylene glycol–water solvent system was chosen due to its wide acceptability in topical formulations, its ability to provide a stable environment for these steroids, and at concentrations above 15% to be self-preserving. From these data there appears to be an approximate tenfold increase in solubility of those steroids which contain the single double bond in the A ring, namely SQ18,566 and SQ20,811, over the two $\Delta^{1,4}$ analogs. The fluorine atom does not seem to be a factor in the solubility of these steroids in the propylene glycol-water system.

The oil-to-water partition coefficients, determined between an aqueous phase containing various propylene glycol–water mixtures and a lipid phase of isopropyl myristate were also determined and these results are shown in Table II. At concentrations of propylene glycol between 30 and 60% the distribution of these steroids is in favor of the lipid phase. When anhydrous propylene glycol was used as the aqueous phase the distribution of these steroids was reversed due to their greater affinity for the glycol phase.

If the stratum corneum can be treated as a lipid containing membrane, then transport of drug from its vehicle into the skin should increase as the lipid partition of the drug is increased. Lipid partitioning together with adequate aqueous solubility in the vehicle should help optimize the effectiveness of topically applied formulations.

Table II. Partition Coefficients of Steroids Between Isopropyl Myristate and Propylene Glycol-Water Mixture. [1]

Compound	Percent Propylene Glycol (w/w)			
	30	40	60	100
SQ 15,361	8.0	6.2	2.0	0.0
SQ 18,566	8.1	5.9	2.6	0.05
SQ 20,589	11.4	6.5	3.6	0.0
SQ 20,811	10.6	6.9	4.8	0.7

[1] at 37°

Table III. Rank Order Activity of Steroid (in Ethanol) Potency using Human Vasoconstrictor and Stripped Skin Assays.

Vasoconstrictor Assay	"Stripped-Skin" Assay
1. SQ 18,566	1. SQ 18,566
2. SQ 15,361	2. SQ 15,361
3. Betamethasone valerate (BMV)	3. Betamethasone valerate
4. SQ 20,589	4. SQ 20,589
5. SQ 20,811	5. SQ 20,811
1 = 2 = 3 =>4 = 5	1 = 2 = 3 = >4 = 5

In the human pharmacological studies, using the vasoconstrictor and stripped skin assays, these four steroids were originally found to be active when applied to the skin as solutions in ethanolic tinctures. The four steroids were further evaluated in a combinatorially designed study using betamethasone valerate as the reference compound and the results of this study are shown in Table III.

In both of these assays, SQ18,566 and SQ15,361 were found to be equal to betamethasone valerate in activity while the two desfluoro analogs, SQ20,589 and SQ20,811, were statistically inferior to the reference steroid.

Table IV. Reversed Passive Arthus Activity of Steroids;
Intradermal and Topical Administration.

| Compound | Average Percent Decrease in Edema | |
	Intradermal (300 γ/site)	Topical[1] (100 mg. cream/site)
Halcinonide (SQ 18,566)	50	43
SQ 20,811	65	40
SQ 20,589	78	20
SQ 15,361	40	19

[1]Six animals per treatment, sites un-occluded.

Currently, both animal and human models are being used to evaluate the efficacy of steroids as formulations. Prior to screening vehicles in humans, the use of the reversed passive Arthus (RPA) assay in rabbits can be utilized. This assay, which uses an immune complex induced reaction, has been shown to be an effective method of assessing anti-inflammatory agents (6). The production of Arthus inflammation is characterized by edema, erythema, hemorrhage and necrosis. Although originally intended to evaluate potential anti-inflammatory agents via the systemic route of administration, topically applied steroid formulations were later used in an attempt to correlate their response with that found in the human vasoconstrictor assay.

The average percent decrease in edema elicited by these four test steroids both by the intradermal route and as topically applied creams is shown in Table IV.

By the intradermal route all four steroids were found to be active in this model, using a baseline of 30% inhibition of edema as being active. However, when topically applied, at a 0.1% concentration in an identical cream base, containing 60% propylene glycol as the solvent system, only SQ18,566 and SQ20,811 were regarded as active formulations. In this study six animals per treatment were used and the sites of application were not occluded. Two of the test steroid creams were further evaluated using the human vasoconstrictor assay. In this study, approximately 40–50 mg of the cream were applied to the sites, which were occluded for 6 hours at which time the occlusive dressing was removed and the area blotted dry. Skin blanching was evaluated at

Table V. Human Vasoconstrictor Assay of Cream Formulations
of Halcinonide (SQ 18,566) and SQ 15,361 as a Function
of Time.[1]

Cream	Occluded Application Percent of Sites Responding At				
	8 hr.	22 hr.	30 hr.	46 hr.	Total
0.1% Halcinonide (SQ 18,566)	89	60	29	6	184
0.1% SQ 15,361	77	54	35	9	175

[1] $N = 28$, 8 sites per patient (4 control, 4 test), double blind.

several time intervals and the data reported in Table V is expressed
as the percent of sites responding at the various time intervals.

Although the two preparations were not found to be statistically different, the data indicate the SQ15,361 cream was less effective than its
Δ^4 analog, SQ18,566. These results are consistent with those found
using the RPA assay and would probably be better exemplified if a
nonoccluded or open technique were used in the human study. The
use of occlusive dressings tends to diminish differences that may exist
between formulations. Each of the four test steroids were further evaluated as 0.1% cream formulations in a double-blind, paired comparison
study in the treatment of hospitalized patients with multiple bilateral
lesions. The creams, each formulated in the same 60% propylene glycol
cream base, were applied three times a day for a maximum of 14 days.
All patients were evaluated daily for evidence of therapeutic response.

The results of this study are shown in Table VI, where a "P" value
of less than 0.05 indicates a statistically significant difference between
the test steroid cream and betamethasone valerate cream. Only halcinonide (SQ18,566) cream was found to be statistically equal to the
reference preparation, while SQ15,361 cream was judged the least effective preparation. The creams containing the two desfluoro analogs,
SQ20,589 and SQ20,811, although not statistically inferior were found
to be less effective than betamethasone valerate cream.

With the exception of SQ15,361, the rank order activity predicted
by the combinatorally designed vasoconstrictor and stripped skin assays
was borne out in this study of therapeutic efficacy.

Table VI. Clinical Responses of Steroid Cream Formulations.

Compound	Test Compound Superior	BMV* Superior	Drug Equal	Neither Drug Effective	Total	Value
SQ 15,361	2	10	7	1	20	0.05
SQ 18,566	8	7	6	0	21	NS**
SQ 20,589	3	11	5	1	20	0.06
SQ 20,811	4	10	6	0	20	0.18

*BMV = betamethasone valerate
**Not Significant

In summary, it appears that the overall biological and physical data generated on these four test steroids indicated that the human vasoconstrictor and stripped assays are appropriate models for assessing the intrinsic activity of steroids and that the intrinsic activity can be lost in a poorly formulated vehicle if steroid solubility and partitioning characteristics are not optimized. In halcinonide cream, approximately 50% of the total concentration of steroid is in solution in the 60% propylene glycol cream vehicle, based on its solubility profile, while the remainder is dispersed as finely micronized crystals. Although SQ15,361 has adequate intrinsic activity, as seen in the ethanolic vasoconstrictor and stripped-skin assays, its poor solubility in the 60% propylene glycol cream vehicle which is approximately one-tenth that of halcinonide seemingly negated its clinical effectiveness.

Similarly, the data obtained from the rabbit model using the Arthus reaction via the topical route appears promising as a preclinical screening assay for formulated topical products.

REFERENCES

1. B.J. Poulsen, Diffusion of drugs from topical vehicles: An analysis of vehicle effects in: "Advances in Biology of Skin," (W. Montagna, R.B. Stoughton, and E.J. Van Scott, eds.), Vol. XII. Meredith, New York, 1972.
2. M. Katz and B.J. Poulsen, Absorption of drugs through the skin, in: "Handbook of Experimental Pharmacology: Concepts in Biochemical Pharmacology" (B.B. Brodie and J.R. Gillette, eds.), Vol. XXVIII/1. Springer-Verlag, New York, 1971.

3. R.J. Scheuplein and I.H. Blank, Permeability of the skin. *Physiol. Rev.* 51, 702–747, (1971).
4. F.K. Bagatell and M.A. Augustine, Evaluation of corticosteroids intended for topical anti-inflammatory drugs. *Curr. Ther. Res.* 16, 748–756 (1974).
5. M.B. Goldlust, D.M. Palner, and M.A. Augustine, Evaluation of topical anti-inflammatory steroid formulations in an Arthus model of inflammation, *J. Inves. Derm.* 66, 157–160 (1976).
6. M.B. Goldlust and W.F. Schreiber, Use of the reversed passive Arthus reaction as a test for anti-inflammatory agents. *Agents and Actions* 5, 39-47 (1975).

Recent Advances in Dermatopharmacology

12

Adrenal Effects of New Topical Steroids

EDWARD C. GOMEZ
LEWIS H. KAMINESTER
PHILLIP FROST

Certain corticosteroids, when topically applied, have been shown to be absorbed through the skin in quantities sufficient to cause effects upon the adrenal-pituitary axis (1,2). In view of the constantly increasing potency of the corticosteroid preparations that are brought to market, the evaluation of the effect of these preparations on the adrenal-pituitary axis is a necessary part of the safety studies done prior to the release of such drugs for general use.

Such investigations have usually consisted of measuring the degree of suppression obtained in patients with normal or diseased skin when large quantities of the formulation under investigation are applied, with or without occlusion, for a relatively short duration of time. Although this methodology might prove to be useful in the selection of steroids that did not cause significant suppression of the adrenal-pituitary axis, the fact is that most steroids currently marketed will, under the conditions of the test, cause adrenal suppression in a very significant number of patients. Since clinically significant effects upon the adrenal–pituitary axis are, in general, more determined by duration of suppression than by the degree of suppression, these studies also do not tell

Halcinonide   Triamcinolone Acetonide   Betamethasone Valerate

1   Chemical structure of corticosteroids.

us the effect of such preparations when used on a more or less continual basis in patients with chronic diseases.

Recently we have had the opportunity to carry out studies intended to investigate the adrenal effects of a new and potent topical corticosteroid, halcinonide, which is marketed by E.R. Squibb and Sons under the name "Halog." We have evaluated the adrenal effects of this formulation both in an acute usage protocol and in a subacute usage protocol which more closely approximates clinical usage.

Halcinonide conforms to the basic chemical structure of earlier halogenated topical corticosteroids in having a fluorine atom in the 9α position and an acetonide linkage at positions 16 and 17 (Fig. 1). It differs from triamcinolone acetonide in that it has a chlorine atom at the 21 position and lacks the double bond at the 1 position.

In view of the reported increase in the efficacy of this new preparation (3), we undertook a study to determine the frequency of adrenal suppression both in a controlled environment where the drug was applied with or without occlusion to normal and diseased skin and when used by outpatients without occlusion in a manner similar to the normal clinical use that might occur in a dermatologist's office. As expected, we found that halcinonide caused reversible adrenal suppression when used with occlusion in patients with psoriasis and caused significant suppression in psoriatics who were treated without occlusion. Normal volunteers treated also showed suppression with occlusion, but not without it.

Table I shows the plasma cortisol values obtained in six patients with extensive psoriasis (greater than 30% of the skin surface involved). Following an initial baseline period, 15 grams of halcinonide cream were applied twice daily to approximately 50% of the body, selecting the

Table I. Effect of Halcinonide Cream on Plasma Cortisol of Psoriatics

Patient	Occlusion	Pretreatment day			Treatment day					Posttreatment day			
		1	2	3	1	2	3	4	5	1	2	3	4
1	No	19.8	24.4	23.6	13.8	16.5	10.2	13.7	9.7	22.5	24.6	22.5	21.7
2	No	19.5	19.5	14.2	11.7	1.4	1.7	5.2	12.6	22.7	21.5	16.4	22.5
3	No	17.6	14.6	—	12.8	17.2	19.1	14.2	11.2	13.2	12.5	12.5	9.4
4	Yes	22.0	19.6	18.7	15.8	17.8	10.5	1.2	2.7	22.2	18.8	17.6	19.7
5	Yes	18.8	25.5	19.5	12.2	9.8	10.4	11.6	3.8	15.4	17.7	15.8	16.2
6	Yes	20.0	29.8	17.6	11.5	4.4	2.5	1.7	1.1	18.7	17.2	24.5	22.1

Units = μg/dl

123

areas most involved with psoriasis. The patients had the treatment areas occluded with Saran Wrap for 10 hours following each application.

Of three patients without occlusion, two had significant lowering of their plasma cortisol levels within 24 hours, one of them having levels of less than 2 μg%. The third patient did not show a significant decrease in plasma cortisol during the five days of treatment. In one of the patients showing decreases in plasma cortisol, the levels of plasma cortisol began to rise back towards normal before cessation of therapy; this was associated with rapid clinical improvement of the lesions.

All three patients treated with occlusion showed decreases of plasma cortisol to low levels by the second day of therapy and all had a rapid return to pretreatment levels the day following the cessation of therapy.

Six normal subjects were similarly treated, three with occlusion and three without (Table II). None of the subjects treated without occlusion had significant decrease in plasma cortisol during therapy, indicating the absence of suppression of adrenal function.

Two of the three normal subjects treated with occlusion showed definite decreases in plasma cortisol levels, which persisted during the treatment period and reversed rapidly on discontinuation of treatment. The third subject showed markedly decreased plasma cortisol only on the fourth treatment day but, although the value obtained that day was extremely low, a technical error cannot be ruled out.

Thus, in the four groups of patients we treated with halcinonide in this acute exposure type of experiment, we found halcinonide with occlusion can induce transient plasma cortisol suppression whether applied to normal or diseased skin.

Without occlusion, one patient showed a profound decrease in plasma cortisol when it was applied to diseased skin and another similar patient showed a moderate, but significant, decrease in plasma cortisol. Application to normal skin without occlusion did not show evidence of absorption sufficient to cause suppression of adrenal function.

In order to compare the results obtained with halcinonide to those with another corticosteroid which has been used clinically, we evaluated the effect of betamethasone valerate (marketed by the Schering Corporation as Valisone) under similar conditions in patients with extensive psoriasis (Table III). Two patients treated with betamethasone valerate cream under occlusion showed a decrease in plasma cortisol levels, with one patient demonstrating a rapid return to normal levels during the treatment period and the second returning to pretreatment values the day following cessation of therapy.

Table II. Effect of Halcinonide Cream on Plasma Cortisol of Normal Subjects

Subject	Occlusion	Pretreatment day			Treatment day					Posttreatment day			
		1	2	3	1	2	3	4	5	1	2	3	4
1	No	26.2	31.3	29.4	27.2	23.1	21.0	22.4	21.7	23.2	25.1	22.4	26.0
2	No	23.8	13.5	21.5	26.5	28.4	29.2	27.8	19.4	25.5	27.3	31.2	22.9
3	No	28.2	27.6	24.6	20.1	24.4	21.0	27.0	29.6	33.2	20.1	33.2	34.0
4	Yes	22.0	25.0	—	21.5	20.5	8.3	6.7	5.9	14.9	22.5	19.5	21.8
5	Yes	26.4	24.6	19.4	14.6	4.6	3.9	2.7	1.9	19.5	22.5	23.5	18.9
6	Yes	8.1	14.3	16.4	15.7	14.7	15.5	1.9	12.8	19.5	18.2	17.6	12.2

Units = μg/dl

Table III. Effect of Betamethasone Valerate Cream on Plasma Cortisol of Psoriatics

Patient	Occlusion	Pretreatment day			Treatment day					Posttreatment day			
		1	2	3	1	2	3	4	5	1	2	3	4
1	No	19.2	15.5	21.5	24.5	15.2	9.5	11.5	16.3	17.2	15.4	18.3	24.5
2	No	29.7	24.5	21.5	19.5	18.7	9.2	8.7	12.5	13.6	12.2	19.4	18.2
3	No	32.3	31.4	10.4	22.5	19.7	17.5	19.9	21.2	18.7	15.4	16.2	22.7
4	Yes	25.4	21.2	19.6	7.3	9.5	14.7	21.5	16.7	18.2	23.6	20.1	19.7
5	Yes	19.8	18.7	17.6	8.6	10.4	8.7	9.5	9.7	18.4	17.6	15.5	16.6

Units = $\mu g/dl$

Table IV. Patients Studied

Number of patients	51
Number completing 4-6 weeks	44
Age	9-76
Male/Female	31/13
% Involvement	1/18 to 9/18
Severity	
severe (no. of patients)	9
moderate (no. of patients)	26
mild (no. of patients)	9
Medication (grams)	225-900 (Avg. = 472)

Treatment of three patients without occlusion resulted in a mild transient decrease in plasma cortisol of one patient, a more pronounced decrease lasting until the second posttreatment day in a second patient, and lack of adrenal effect in a third patient.

These data indicate that both halcinonide cream and betamethasone valerate cause decrease of plasma cortisol levels when applied with occlusion to patients with widespread psoriasis. Without occlusion, halcinonide caused significant decrease of plasma cortisol in two of three patients with widespread psoriasis, while betamethasone valerate caused less pronounced decreases in one, or possibly two, out of three patients. Halcinonide also caused decrease in plasma cortisol of normal subjects when administered under occlusion, but not without occlusion.

The second phase of our study was based on the clinical use of these topical corticosteroids in a group of outpatients in a manner similar to that most dermatologists would use in treating a wide variety of skin disorders, except, of course, that these patients had access to liberal amounts of the creams, supplied without charge.

Of 51 patients with psoriasis enrolled in the study, 44 completed a treatment regimen of from 4 to 6 weeks of t.i.d. topical application without occlusion. Patients were assigned to either betamethasone valerate (Valisone) or halcinonide (Halog) in a double-blind randomized manner and seen at weekly intervals for objective determination of their clinical response. Plasma cortisol levels were determined weekly. Patients were seen at the same time of day on each visit to minimize the effect of diurnal variation of cortisol production.

As shown in Table IV, the patients completing the study ranged from 9 to 76 years of age, there being 13 women and 31 men. The

Table V. Summary of Results of Subacute Usage Study

	Halog	Valisone
Number of patients	23	21
Adrenal suppression[a]	2	0
Striae formation[a]	3	0
Clinical response[a]		
excellent	13 (57%)	1 (4%)
good	3 (13%)	12 (57%)
fair	4 (17%)	6 (29%)
poor	3 (13%)	2 (10%)

[a]Number of patients with.

average amount of cream used by each patient was 472 gm, with a range of from 225 to 900 gm. Involvement varied from 5% of the body surface to more than 50% involvement.

Of the 44 patients, 9 had mild involvement, 26 had moderate, and 9 had severe involvement. The clinical and laboratory responses noted are summarized in Table V.

Of the 44 patients completing the period of therapy, only two showed definite decreases in plasma cortisol (Table V); both of these patients were in the halcinonide treatment group. Table VI shows the data for these two patients.

The first patient was a 72 year old woman with psoriasis of moderate severity, involving the arms, scalp, trunk, legs, and groin (about 5% total surface area). She completed four weeks of therapy with an overall excellent response. Baseline plasma cortisol levels were 17 μg%, whereas cortisol levels during treatment varied from 4 to 9 μg%. Three weeks following therapy a follow-up cortisol determination was 17 μg%.

The second patient was a 70-year-old man with psoriasis of moderate severity, involving areas of the face, neck, arms, scalp, trunk, buttocks, groin, and feet (about 10% of the total surface area). He had a baseline cortisol level of 21 μg%. Except for the first week of therapy, all his cortisol levels were below 10 μg%. A follow-up cortisol level, 7 weeks after termination of therapy, was 17 μg%. This man also showed an overall excellent clinical response.

It is interesting to note that neither of these patients were among the most involved, either in severity of psoriasis, or in the amount of surface area involved. Neither had any noteworthy side effects.

Table VI. Patients Showing Adrenal Suppression
in Subacute Usage Study

| | Plasma Cortisol level (μg/dl)[a] | |
	P.S.	M.L.
Pretreatment	20.7	18.4
Treatment		
1 week	13.1	4.5
2 weeks	8.8	8.4
3 weeks	8.7	9.5
4 weeks	10.2	5.9
5 weeks	5.7	−
6 weeks	7.7	−
Posttreatment		
3 weeks	−	17.6
7 weeks	17.2	−

[a]Average of two blood specimens drawn at each visit.

The only side effect noted during this study was the formation of striae in three patients, all of whom were in the group treated with halcinonide (Table V). The striae were in areas of natural occlusion, except for one patient who developed striae encircling the waist, corresponding to the area of a wide leather belt which he customarily wore.

The concentration of the effects noted in the halcinonide group is not surprising since the efficacy data (Table V) indicates that halcinonide had greater clinical efficacy than betamethasone valerate.

The adrenal suppression observed in the acute usage studies with patients having widespread psoriasis is consistent with the findings in previous studies with other steroid preparations. No adrenal effects were noted when halcinonide was applied to the skin of normal subjects unless the area was occluded.

In the outpatient study only two of 22 psoriatics using halcinonide without occlusion showed a definite pattern of adrenal suppression. None of the patients treated with betamethasone valerate showed suppression. Thus, the number of patients showing suppression in this second phase of our investigation contrasts with the previous findings in the acute usage study. The conditions of exposure differed considerably in that (a) only 5% involvement of the body surface was required for patient selection, (b) the use of the medication was not supervised by nursing personnel, (c) the time of evaluation and cortisol determination differed in that the first sampling occurred after a longer period of usage (1 week) than the entire treatment period in the inpatient study, and (d) sufficient time elapsed for greater clinical improvement of the lesions. The results obtained were surprising in that the only two patients who showed mild reversible adrenal suppression in the outpatient study were not among the most involved psoriatics, having only 5–10% involvement, and both showed excellent clinical response by the end of treatment period. Both were elderly individuals and may have differed from the other patients in adrenal–pituitary reserve rather than in amount of exposure to the medication.

Because of the differing time course of the protocols, patients in the outpatient study may have had transient decreases in plasma cortisol and returned to their normal levels prior to the first evaluation after 1 week of therapy.

We feel that the subacute-usage type of study is probably of more value than the acute-usage study in predicting adrenal problems likely to be encountered in clinical practice, since it more closely simulates this situation. The potency of present day topical steroid preparations makes studies involving application to diseased skin in large amounts or with occlusion of limited value since it is expected that most patients will show suppression under these circumstances.

If it is desired to determine whether new formulations will present more problems with regards to effects on the adrenal–pituitary axis when topically applied, it would be more meaningful to conduct the studies using normal subjects, with and without occlusion, since the suppression of adrenal function would be a better guide of potential hazard in clinical usage. Since diminution of adrenal-pituitary reserve is more a function of the duration of suppression than of degree (low daily dose corticosteroid therapy over a long period of time results in greater impairment than large doses for a short period), the evaluation of new formulations by outpatient studies lasting 6 weeks or longer will be more meaningful, as regards the hazards of the new formulation when applied to diseased skin. Since such studies can easily be combined with early pilot studies of efficacy, they will provide data concerning adrenal effects early in the evaluation of the new preparation as well as reduce the development cost which must ultimately be passed on to the consumer.

REFERENCES

1. R.B. Scoggins, and A.L. Kligman, Percutaneous absorption of cortico-steroid. *N. Engl. J. Med.* 173, 831–840 (1965).
2. R.D. Carr and W.M. Baxter, Percutaneous absorption of corticosteroids. Adrenal cortical suppression with total body induction. *Acta. Derm-venerol.* 48, 417–428 (1968).
3. E. Leibshim and F.K. Bagatell, Halcinonide in the treatment of cortico-steroid responsive dermatoses. *Brit. J. Dermatol.* 90, 435–440 (1974).

Recent Advances in Dermatopharmacology

13

Topical Nonsteroidal Antiinflammatory Agents

RONALD J. TRANCIK

I. INTRODUCTION

The discovery in the early 1970's that aspirin-like drugs inhibit prostaglandin biosynthesis led to an explosive research effort to support the concept that the mode of action of nonsteroidal antiinflammatory drugs was related to the blockade of prostaglandin biosynthesis. This burgeoning research activity has been extensively reviewed (1). The role of prostaglandins in cutaneous biology and inflammation has also been discussed in detail (2-4). The purpose of this chapter is to present a brief overview of several aspects of dermatopharmacological research on nonsteroidal antiinflammatory drugs. Recent studies describing topical application of these drugs on guinea pigs and man will be presented. Inhibition of prostaglandin synthesis by several nonsteroidal antiinflammatory agents and a receptor site theory, which has been proposed as a unifying concept to describe the mechanism of action of nonsteroidal antiinflammatory agents, will also be discussed.

Table I. Effect of Nonsteroidal Antiinflammatory Agents on
Prostaglandin Synthetase

Compound	Concentration [M]	Percent inhibition	Relative activity
Mefenamic acid	5×10^{-5}	100	
	5×10^{-6}	97	12.1
Diflumidone	5×10^{-5}	100	
	5×10^{-6}	95	11.9
Indomethacin	5×10^{-5}	100	
	5×10^{-6}	84	10.5
Flufenamic acid	5×10^{-5}	93	
	5×10^{-6}	53	6.6
Phenylbutazone	5×10^{-5}	81	
	5×10^{-6}	22	2.8
Bufexamac	5×10^{-5}	18	
	5×10^{-6}	12	1.5
Ibuprofen	5×10^{-5}	61	
	5×10^{-6}	11	1.4
Aspirin	5×10^{-5}	9	
	5×10^{-6}	8	1.0

II. LABORATORY STUDIES

A. Inhibition of Prostaglandin Synthesis

Prostaglandins have been implicated as mediators of several different types of inflammatory skin reactions (4). Prostaglandins and prostaglandin-like substances have been isolated from perfusates of skin after ultraviolet light induced inflammation, contact dermatitis, or thermal burns (5). Drugs such as aspirin and indomethacin have been found to inhibit prostaglandin synthesis in skin (6,7). This property may explain the activity of nonsteroidal antiinflammatory agents.

The inhibitory effects and relative activities of several nonsteroidal antiinflammatory agents on prostaglandin synthetase are summarized in Table I (8,9). The results obtained with the reference agents are

Table II. Dose Related Effect of Diflumidone and Indomethacin
on Prostaglandin Synthetase

Compound	Concentration [M]	Percent inhibition
Diflumidone	5×10^{-5}	100
	5×10^{-6}	95
	2×10^{-7}	73
	1×10^{-7}	64
Indomethacin	5×10^{-5}	100
	5×10^{-6}	84
	2×10^{-7}	17
	1×10^{-7}	15
Diflumidone +	2×10^{-7}	93
indomethacin	1×10^{-7}	84

consistent with those reported by Flower et al. (6,7). Two relatively new compounds, diflumidone (3-benzoyldifluoromethanesulfonanilide) and bufexamac (p-butoxyphenylacethydroxamic acid), are also included in Table I. Diflumidone is a unique, acidic nonsteroidal antiinflammatory agent and its chemistry and systemic pharmacology have been reported (10,11). The use of bufexamac on diseased skin is discussed later in this chapter.

The molar [M] concentrations of diflumidone and indomethacin were reduced in an attempt to determine the minimum inhibitory concentration on the prostaglandin synthetase system (Table II) (9). At lower concentrations (10^{-7} M), diflumidone was found to be more inhibitory than indomethacin. When diflumidone and indomethacin were combined, an additive inhibitory effect on prostaglandin synthetase was observed (Table II). This suggests that the two molecules may be operating by the same mechanism.

The data in Tables I and II were obtained by the method of White and Glassman (12) which involves measuring prostaglandin synthetase activity by radiochemically determining the conversion of ^{3}H-arachidonic acid into prostaglandin E_2 and $F_{2\alpha}$. The enzyme was isolated from microsomal extracts of bovine seminal vesicles. Nonsteroidal antiinflammatory agents were dissolved in buffer solution or 50% methanol and their ability to inhibit prostaglandin synthetase at various concentrations determined.

Table III. Effect of Topical Diflumidone and Reference Agents in Plastibase®
On UV Erythema of Guinea Pig Skin

Treatment	Concentration (%)	Average score/ animal ± se	Protected/ used	Percent protected
Diflumidone	5.0	1.9 ± 0.6	7/7	100
	2.0	1.3 ± 0.5	13/14	93
	1.0	3.1 ± 0.7	9/14	64
	0.5	2.9 ± 1.0	5/7	71
	0.1	5.1 ± 0.7	2/7	29
Indomethacin	3.0	0	6/6	100
	2.0	6.6 ± 1.1	1/7	14
	1.0	7.3 ± 0.5	0/7	0
Aspirin	5.0	6.3 ± 0.7	2/7	29
Phenylbutazone	5.0	5.1 ± 0.6	3/7	43
Hydrocortisone	3.0	7.2 ± 0.4	0/10	0
Vehicle (Plastibase®)	–	7.4 ± 0.3	2/28	7

The inhibitory effect of corticosteroids on the prostaglandin synthetase system is controversial. Although corticosteroids are among the
most potent antiinflammatory agents available, they were found to
lack inhibitory effects on prostaglandin synthesis in several systems
(6,13). Lewis and Piper (14) suggested that the action of corticoids
in inflammation results from inhibition of release, but not synthesis,
of prostaglandins. More recently, it has been shown that corticosteroids
do inhibit prostaglandin formation in cell culture systems (15,16).

B. Inhibition of UV-Induced Erythema in Guinea Pigs

Topical nonsteroidal and steroidal antiinflammatory agents have
been studied in the guinea pig after UV-induced erythema. Lambelin
et al. (17,18), found that bufexamac applied topically was more active
than either phenylbutazone or aspirin and that fluocinolone acetonide
was inactive. Snyder and Eaglstein (19) reported that *intradermal* indomethacin was approximately 45 times more effective than aspirin in

Table IV. Effect of Topical Diflumidone and Reference Agents in Solution
On UV Erythema of Guinea Pig Skin

Treatment	Concentration (%)	Average score/ animal ± se	Protected/ used	Percent protected
Diflumidone	4.0	0.6 ± 0.6	5/5	100
	2.5	0	5/5	100
	1.0	1.0 ± 0.8	4/4	100
Indomethacin	4.0	1.0 ± 0.6	4/4	100
	2.5	0	5/5	100
	1.0	1.0 ± 0.7	4/4	100
Aspirin	4.0	5.3 ± 1.5	1/4	25
	1.0	6.8 ± 0.4	0/5	0
Hydrocortisone	4.0	7.2 ± 0.6	0/5	0
	1.0	8.0 ± 0.4	0/4	0
Vehicle (PG:EtOH:DMA, 19:19:2 v/v)	–	8.4 ± 0.2	0/10	0

reducing erythema in guinea pigs and that both triamcinolone acetonide and hydrocortisone were inactive. Snyder (20) later described a marked decrease in UV-induced erythema in guinea pigs following *topical* application of indomethacin.

Tables III, IV, and V summarize the effect of diflumidone and other antiinflammatory drugs on UV-induced erythema in guinea pigs when applied topically either as ointment suspensions (Plastibase®) or solutions immediately after irradiation (21). The method of Winder et al. (22), with minor modifications was used. Materials were applied to a region of depilated skin of fasted male guinea pigs immediately after exposure of this region to ultraviolet light. Three exposed circular areas of skin on the ventrolateral surface of each animal were scored 2 hours after exposure. Each erythema was scored separately on a 0 to +3 scale and the total score for each animal was recorded (maximum score/animal = 9). The percentage of guinea pigs protected from developing erythema, those with total scores less than 5, was determined. Treatments were randomized and the scorer was not aware of the treatment any animal had received.

Table V. Effect of Topical Diflumidone and Indomethacin in Propylene Glycol
On UV Erythema of Guinea Pig Skin

Treatment	Concentration (%)	Average score/ animal ± se	Protected/ used	Percent protected
Diflumidone	8.0	0.1 ± 0.1	7/7	100
	2.0	1.4 ± 0.9	6/7	86
	0.5	4.6 ± 1.5	3/7	43
Indomethacin	2.0	4.1 ± 1.1	4/7	57
Vehicle (Propylene Glycol)	—	8.3 ± 0.5	0/7	0

When drugs were applied as Plastibase® suspensions (Table III), diflumidone and indomethacin were markedly more effective than aspirin or phenylbutazone and hydrocortisone was inactive. The concentration of diflumidone required to protect 50% of the animals from developing erythema can be estimated from Table III to be approximately 0.3%. At comparable concentrations in Plastibase®, diflumidone was found to be more potent than indomethacin.

The effect of antiinflammatory agents after solubilization in the vehicle reported by Snyder and Eaglstein (23) is shown in Table IV. Again, diflumidone and indomethacin exhibited high levels of activity whereas aspirin and hydrocortisone showed little or no activity. A comparison of the activities of diflumidone and indomethacin in propylene glycol solution is summarized in Table V. In solution, diflumidone and indomethacin appear equipotent in their ability to inhibit the UV-induced erythema in guinea pigs.

The important role that vehicles play in dermatopharmacological evaluations is becoming increasingly evident (24). It is interesting to note the vehicle effect observed in the present study. For example, 1% indomethacin in solution (Table IV) gave 100% inhibition of erythema, whereas, when formulated in the Plastibase® ointment at the same concentration (Table III), there was no protection. Likewise, 1% diflumidone in solution compared to ointment gave 100% and 64% protection, respectively. Smaller differences in activity, which can be attributed to differences in the solution vehicles, are also apparent from the data contained in Tables IV and V.

When evaluating topically applied agents as inhibitors of UV-induced erythema, it is important to realize that they, or the vehicles in which they are formulated, may absorb a significant amount of UV light when applied *prior* to irradiation. Such compounds may not be acting as antiinflammatories but rather as UV screening agents. For example, it was reported that hydrocortisone would delay UV-induced erythema in guinea pigs when applied before, but not after, irradiation (25). Hydrocortisone has an absorption maxima at 242 nm and, depending upon the light source used in the study, can act as an effective UV-light screening agent (26).

III. CLINICAL STUDIES

A. Inhibition of UV-Induced Erythema in Man

Snyder and Eaglstein (19) found that indomethacin, aspirin, and triamcinolone acetonide decreased and delayed UV-induced erythema when injected *intradermally* in humans. The same investigators described a marked decrease in erythema when indomethacin was applied *topically* (23). Topical fluocinonide, however, was no better than the vehicle control. This was expected since at exposures greater than one minimal erythemal dose, effects of corticosteroids on UV-induced erythema in human skin are difficult to demonstrate (27,28). Snyder (20) reported that epidermal responses to UV injury such as keratinocyte cell death and altered DNA synthesis proceeded unmodified after topical application of indomethacin. Eaglstein (29) has indicated that the concept of a nonsteroidal antiinflammatory agent such as indomethacin being useful in inflammatory dermatologic conditions by inhibiting prostaglandin synthesis is exciting; however, current data are insufficient to justify the conclusion that indomethacin is either effective or safe for use in sunburn.

An important experimental detail to consider when conducting inhibition of UV-induced erythema evaluations was pointed out by Eaglstein and Marsico (30). They found that intradermal doses of indomethacin, which were effective antagonists of UV-B (280–320 nm) induced erythema, had little effect on erythema induced by UV-C (predominately 250 nm) light. It was suggested that this result was consistent with the possibility that the prostaglandins participate in UV-B but not UV-C induced inflammation.

B. Bufexamac

Reports in the dermatological literature on the use of nonsteroidal antiinflammatory agents on diseased skin are sparse; although, some clinical and pharmacological data are available on bufexamac. In a review published in 1974, it was concluded that bufexamac has definite antiinflammatory activity, but data on its efficacy were insufficient to show whether there are circumstances in which it has advantages over corticosteroids (31). Several additional clinical studies of bufexamac have since appeared and are mentioned below.

In a double blind, parallel clinical study of 4 weeks duration, no difference was found between bufexamac cream and fluocinolone ace-tonide cream in their effect on various dermatoses (32). The majority of the patients had contact dermatitis and there were no psoriatics in this study.

In a double blind, bilateral comparison, bufexamac ointment was evaluated against a placebo ointment in a study lasting 10 days (33). Bufexamac was found to be superior to its vehicle. Only patients with psoriasis were included; however, they were pretreated for 5 days with a 5% salicylic acid ointment.

In an open study, the use of bufexamac cream in the treatment of a typical cross section of dermatologic conditions seen in general prac-tice was evaluated (34). The majority of the patients were diagnosed as having contact dermatitis, pruritis, or eczema mostly of mild severity. When the condition was moderately severe or severe, the cure rate was lower. It was concluded that bufexamac cream has a place in the man-agement of a wide range of common skin disorders.

In a comparative study, bufexamac and two corticosteroid creams were evaluated (35). A double blind, bilateral, 4 week design was utilized which compared bufexamac to either betamethasone-17-valerate or fluocinolone acetonide. Diagnoses were eczema, contact dermatitis, and allergic contact dermatitis. The investigators concluded that similar results were obtained with bufexamac and betamethasone-17-valerate, and although the results were slightly better with fluocinolone acetonide, the differences were not statistically significant.

Based on available clinical data, bufexamac appears to be effective in many of the steroid responsive dermatoses with the notable exception of psoriasis. Most of the clinical trials with bufexamac reported to date, however, utilize skin diseases, such as irritant or allergic contact derma-titis, which are self-limiting and will remit either spontaneously or upon removal of the challenge agent. Additional definitive clinical data on the use of bufexamac in psoriasis and other dermatologic conditions are needed.

IV. RECEPTOR-SITE THEORY

A hypothetical receptor site for classical antiinflammatory agents was proposed a number of years ago and has been discussed in detail (36,37). The theory was based on structure activity relationships in a number of chemical series (i.e., indomethacin, aspirin, phenylbutazone, anthranilic acids) and on the assumption that classical antiinflammatory agents acted at the same site. The two primary features of this "cloverleaf" receptor site, a trough to accept a twisted ring and a cationic site which allows binding of the carboxylic anion, are depicted in Fig. 1.

As a result of studying molecular models, it was visualized that prostaglandins closely resemble indomethacin, and other classical non-steroidal antiinflammatory agents, in the conformation shown in Fig. 2. It has been proposed that the role of the receptor is to hold the unsaturated fatty acid, arachidonic acid, in proper orientation and that the trough is where oxygenation-cyclization of arachidonic acid occurs to form prostaglandins E_2 and $F_{2\alpha}$ (36). In other words, the receptor site can be thought of as the prostaglandin synthetase enzyme system. Since many of the nonsteroidal antiinflammatory agents are highly active and specific in inhibiting prostaglandin synthesis, it has been proposed that these agents are competitively inhibiting formation of prostaglandins by effectively competing for the receptor site.

This hypothetical receptor site has been employed as a unifying concept by investigators working in inflammation research. Further study into the mode of action of classical and nonclassical antiinflammatory agents *in vivo* should lead to a better understanding of the receptor site theory.

V. CONCLUSIONS

Many of the classical nonsteroidal antiinflammatory agents are potent inhibitors of prostaglandin biosynthesis *in vitro*. It has been found that these compounds also inhibit and delay the formation of UV-induced erythema in both man and guinea pigs. Consequently, this has led some investigators to propose prostaglandins as mediators of cutaneous inflammation. These findings may have profound clinical sig-

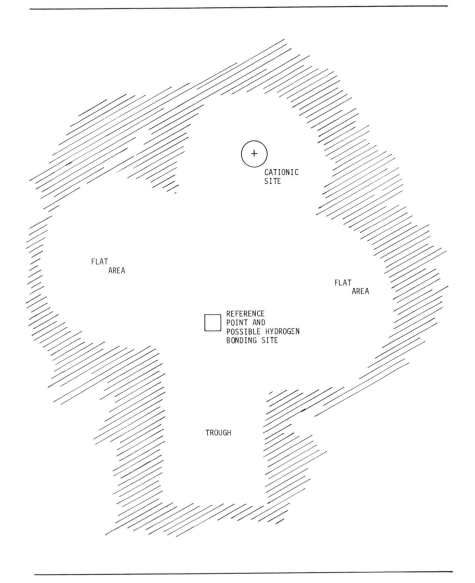

CATIONIC
SITE

FLAT
AREA

FLAT
AREA

REFERENCE
POINT AND
POSSIBLE HYDROGEN
BONDING SITE

TROUGH

1 A hypothetical receptor site derived by considering the molecular spacial requirements and orientations of classical nonsteroidal antiinflammatory agents (from reference 36; with permission).

2

A possible conformation of PGE$_2$ at the prostaglandin synthetase antiinflammatory receptor compared with indomethacin, a potent inhibitor (from reference 36; with permission).

nificance in dermatology and ultimately lead to compounds which may be used in the treatment of cutaneous inflammatory diseases. To date, however, bufexamac is the only topical nonsteroidal antiinflammatory agent currently on the market and is not available in the United States.

Two objectives of conducting research in this area are to uncover new, active molecules and to study the mechanism of the inflammatory response. It is interesting to note that the latter objective has led to the discovery of a new series of cellular regulatory agents and that the roles of prostaglandins should now be re-examined in light of this recent discovery. These new regulators, thromboxanes, have been isolated and have half-lives on the order of 30 seconds but are, in some cases, hundreds of time more potent than prostaglandins (38). Figure 3 outlines the conversion of arachidonic acid to endoperoxide (PGG$_2$) which can then be converted to PGE$_2$ and PGF$_{2\alpha}$ or follow an alternate pathway to form thromboxanes (A$_2$ and B$_2$). The mode of action of these

3   Conversion of arachidonic acid to endoperoxide (PGG$_2$) which can then undergo transformation to either prostaglandins (PGE$_2$ and PGF$_2\alpha$) or thromboxanes (A$_2$ and B$_2$).

cellular mediators should be better understood within the next few years. This active area of research should also uncover the clinical and biological roles of these cellular mediators and may better define the clinical use of topical nonsteroidal antiinflammatory agents in dermatology.

ACKNOWLEDGMENTS

K.F. Swingle, Ph.D., R.L. Vigdahl, Ph.D., and R.A. Scherrer, Ph.D., of Riker Laboratories, Inc. are gratefullly acknowledged for their contributions to this chapter.

REFERENCES

1. H.J. Robinson, J.R. Vane (eds.), "Prostaglandin Synthetase Inhibitors— Their Effects on Physiological Functions and Pathological States." Raven Press, New York, 1974.
2. R. Kumar, L.M. Solomon, Prostaglandins in cutaneous biology. *Arch Dermatol.* 106, 101–107 (1972).
3. V.A. Ziboh, Prostaglandins and their biological significance in the skin. *Int. J. Dermatol.* 14, 485–493 (1975).
4. M.E. Goldyne, Prostaglandins and cutaneous inflammation. *J. Invest. Dermatol.* 64, 377–385 (1975).
5. M.W. Greaves, W. McDonald-Gibson, Effect of non-steroidal antiinflammatory and antipyretic drugs on prostaglandin biosynthesis by human skin. *J. Invest. Dermatol.* 61, 127–129 (1973).
6. R.J. Flower, R. Gryglewski, K. Herbaczynska-Cedro, J.R. Vane, Effects of antiinflammatory drugs on prostaglandin biosynthesis. *Nature [New Biol.]* 238, 104–106 (1972).
7. R.J. Flower, H.C. Cheung, D.W. Cushman, Quantitative determination of prostaglandins and malondialdhyde formed by the arachidonate oxygenase (prostaglandin synthetase) system of bovine seminal vescile. *Prostaglandins* 4, 325–341 (1973).
8. R.L. Vigdahl, R.H. Tukey, Mechanism of action of novel antiinflammatory drugs diflumidone and R-805. *Pharmacologist* 17, 226 (1975).
9. R.L. Vigdahl, unpublished data.
10. J.K.Harrington, J.E. Robertson, D.C. Kvam, R.R. Hamilton, K.T. McGurran, R.J. Trancik, K.F. Swingle, G.G.I. Moore, J.F. Gerster, Antiinflammatory agents. I. 3-Benzoylfluoroalkanesulfonanilides. *J. Med. Chem.* 13, 137 (1970).
11. K.F. Swingle, R.R. Hamilton, J.K. Harrington, D.C. Kvam, 3-Benzoyldifluoromethanesulfonanilide, sodium salt (diflumidone sodium MBR 4164–8): A new antiinflammatory agent. *Arch. Int. Pharmacodyn. Ther.* 189, 129–144 (1971).
12. H.L. White, A.T. Glassman, A simple radiochemical assay for prostaglandin synthetase. *Prostaglandins* 7, 123–129 (1974).
13. J.R. Vane, Inhibition of prostaglandin synthesis as a mechanism of action for aspirin-like drugs. *Nature [New Biol]* 231, 232–235 (1971).

14. G.P. Lewis, P.J. Piper, Inhibition of release of prostaglandins as an explanation of some of the actions of anti-inflammatory corticosteroids. *Nature (London)* 254, 308–311, 1975.
15. F. Kantrowitz, D.R. Robinson, M.B. McGuire, L. Levine, Corticosteroids inhibit prostaglandin production by rheumatoid synovia. *Nature (London)* 258, 737–739 (1975).
16. A.H. Tashjian, E.F. Voelkel, J. McDonough, L. Levine, Hydrocortisone inhibits prostaglandin production by mouse fibrosarcoma cells. *Nature (London)* 258, 739–741 (1975).
17. G. Lambelin, D. Vassart-Thys, J. Roba, Pharmacological studies of bufexamac topically applied on the skin. *Arch. Int. Pharmacodyn. Ther.* 187, 401–414 (1970).
18. G. Lambelin, D. Vassart-Thys, J. Roba, Cutaneous thermometry for topical therapy evaluation of U.V. erythema in the guinea-pig. *Arzneim Forsch.* 21, 44–47 (1971).
19. D.S. Snyder, W.H. Eaglstein, Intradermal anti-prostaglandin agents and sunburn. *J. Invest. Dermatol.* 62, 47–50 (1974).
20. D.S. Snyder, Cutaneous effects of topical indomethacin, an inhibitor of prostaglandin synthesis, on UV-damaged skin. *J. Invest. Dermatol.* 64, 322-325 (1975).
21. K.F. Swingle, Unpublished data.
22. C.V. Winder, J. Wax, V. Burr, M. Been, C.E. Rosiere, A study of pharmacological influences on ultraviolet erythema in guinea pigs. *Arch. Int. Pharmacodyn. Ther.* 116, 261–292 (1958).
23. D.S. Snyder, W.H. Eaglstein, Topical indomethacin and sunburn. *Br. J. Dermatol.* 90, 91–93 (1974).
24. K.H. Kaidbey, A.M. Kligman, Topical photosensitizers. *Arch. Dermatol.* 110, 868–870 (1974).
25. M.L. Graeme, P. Peters, K. Maiorana, C. Cooper, The effect of topically applied agents on ultraviolet erythema in guinea pigs. *Pharmacologist* 17, 226 (1975).
26. N.B. Kanof, Observations on the effects of local application of hydrocortisone upon thermal burns and ultraviolet erythema. *J. Invest. Dermatol.* 25, 329–334 (1955).
27. K.H. Burdick, J.K. Haleblain, B.J. Poulsen, S.E. Cobner, Corticosteroid ointments: comparison by two biassays. *Curr. Ther. Res.* 15, 233–242 (1973).
28. K.H. Kaidbey, A.M. Kligman, Assay of topical corticosteroids by suppression of experimental inflammation in humans. *J. Invest. Dermatol.* 63, 292–297 (1974).
29. W.H. Eaglstein, Indomethacin: treatment for sunburn or investigative tool in ultraviolet light inflammation? *Int. J. Dermatol.* 14, 501–502 (1975).
30. W.H. Eaglstein, A.R. Marsico, Dichotomy in response to indomethacin

in UV-C and UV-B induced ultraviolet light inflammation. *J. Invest. Dermatol.* 65, 238–240 (1975).

31. M.B. Herxheimer (ed.), Parfenac. *Drug and Therapeutics Bulletin* 12, 102–103 (1974).
32. J.P. Mackey, A double-blind clinical study of bufexamac and fluocinolone acetonide in dermatitis. *J. Irish Med. Assoc.* 67, 214–216 (1974).
33. J. Van Der Meersch, Comparative study of bufexamac (Droxaryl) ointment and of its excipient on psoriasis cases: double-blind test. *Curr. Ther. Res.* 16, 904–908 (1974).
34. J.C. Valle-Jones, Bufexamac in the treatment of skin diseases in general practice. *Practitioner* 213, 383–386 (1974).
35. D. Wheatley (coord.), A non-steroidal anti-inflammatory cream. A report from the general practitioner research group. *Practitioner* 214, 689-692 (1975).
36. R.A. Scherrer, Introduction to the chemistry of antiinflammatory and antiarthritic agents, *in* R.A. Scherrer and M.W. Whitehouse (eds.), "Antiinflammatory Agents," Vol. 1, pp. 29–43. Academic Press, New York. 1974.
37. T.Y. Shen, E.A. Ham, V.J. Cirillo, M. Zanetti, Structure–activity relationships of certain prostaglandin synthetase inhibitors, *in* H.J. Robinson and J.R. Vane (eds.), "Prostaglandin Synthetase Inhibitors—Their Effects on Physiological Functions and Pathological States," pp. 19–31. Raven Press, New York. 1974.
38. G.B. Kolata, Thromboxanes: The power behind prostaglandins? *Science* 190, 770–771, 812 (1975).

Recent Advances in Dermatopharmacology

14

Thalidomide for Polymorphous Light-Like Eruptions in American Indians

FABIO LONDOÑO

In many countries of Latin America (Fig. 1) a kind of chronic polymorphous light eruption which attacks the lower social classes is frequently seen. It has familial incidence (Fig. 2), begins early in childhood, and has a very long course without significant remissions (often throughout the entire life of the patient). In addition to the usual areas of involvement in light related disease, such as the face, posterior neck, and extensor surfaces of the extremities (Fig. 3), these patients have frequent involvement of the lower lip (Fig. 4) and conjunctiva (Fig. 5).

The skin lesions in these patients seem to combine the plaque-like, prurigo-like, and eczematous forms of chronic polymorphous light eruption. These characteristics have led many Latin American workers (Fig. 6) to segregate it from the classical chronic polymorphous light eruption, resulting in a varied nomenclature (prurigo de Verano, prurigo actinico, erupcion polimorfa a la Luz, dermatitis solar, prurigo solar, and sindrome cutaneo Guatemalense (1-5). In our work we have used the name prurigo actinico in describing this disease.

Since 1960, North American workers have called attention to the high incidence of a special form of solar dermatitis among North Ameri-

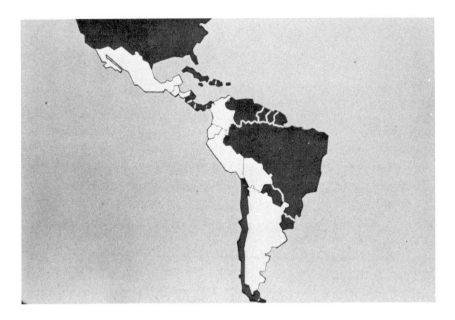

1   Distribution of actinic prurigo in South America, Central America, and Mexico.

can Indian groups (Fig. 7). Schenck (6) reported dermatitis actinica occurring in 13 members of the Chippewa tribe in Minnesota, and Everett et al. (7) reported seven cases of polymorphic light-sensitivity occurring in full-blooded Indians of various tribes in Oklahoma. The clinical and evolutionary characteristics, as well as the histological findings are comparable to those described in the Latin American literature. More recently Birt (8) published 64 cases with the same characteristics in Manitoba Indians. On learning of our work (9) concerning "Familial Actinic Prurigo" he reviewed our material and published a comparison of his cases with ours, in which he concludes that they constitute the same disease and postulates that it may be transmitted as an autosomal dominant trait (10). We agree with Birt and believe the high incidence of the disease in the lower social economic classes of Latin America is due to the relatively high incidence of Indian blood in this group. Figure 8 shows a comparison of one of our cases to that of Birt occurring in a North American Indian.

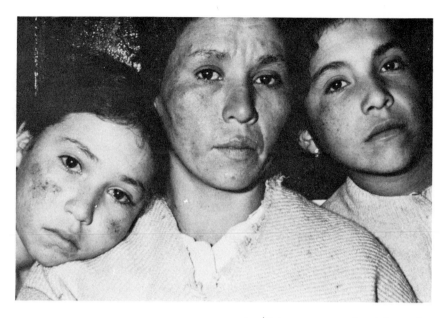

2 Familial occurrence of actinic prurigo.

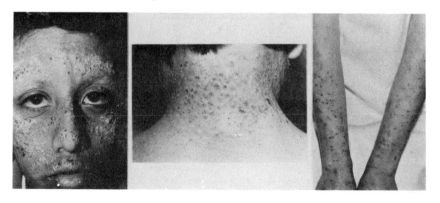

3 Photodistribution of actinic prurigo.

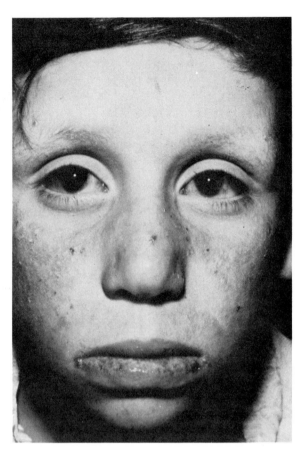

4   Patient with actinic prurlgo demonstrating cholitis of the lower lip.

On the basis of questionnaires sent to all the members of the American Medical Association, requesting information about this disease among American Indians, Birt prepared a map which shows that the geographical distribution of this photodermatitis in North American Indians is confined to the Central Plains of Canada and the United States (Fig. 9).

The pathogenetic mechanisms of this disease remain obscure and, due to its chronic nature and severity, constitutes a considerable clinical

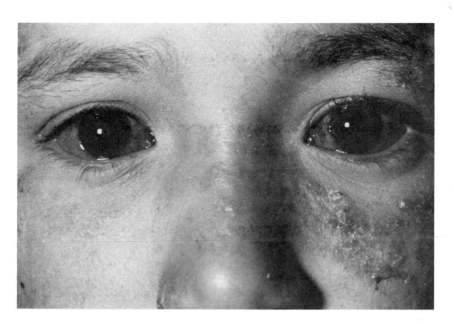

5 Patient with actinic prurigo demonstrating conjunctavitis.

LATIN AMERICA NOMENCLATURE			
PRURIGO SOLAR	López González	Argentina	1952
PRURIGO ACTINICO	Fabio Londoño	Colombia	1961
ECZEMA SOLAR	González Ochoa	México	1962
DERMATITIS SOLAR	Malacara	México	1962
DERMATITIS POLIMORFA A LA LUZ	Corrales Padilla	Honduras	1971
SINDROME CUTANEO GUATEMALENSE	Cordero	Guatemala	1971

6 Latin American nomenclature.

NORTH AMERICAN AND CANADIAN NOMENCLATURE			
SOLAR DERMATITIS OF CHIPEWA INDIANS	SHENCK	U.S.A.	1960
LIGHT SENSITIVE ERUPTION IN AMERICAN INDIANS	EVERETT	U.S.A.	1961
PHOTODERMATITIS IN INDIANS OF MANITOBA	BIRT	CANADA	1968

7   North American and Canadian nomenclature.

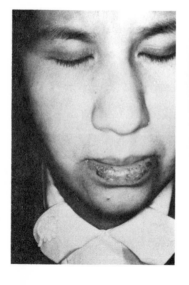
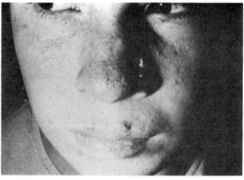

8   Similarity between the North American and South American diseases. Left: North American Indian patient. Right: South American Indian patient.

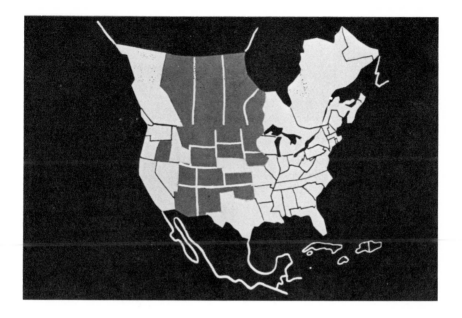

9

Geographical distribution of photodermatitis in North American Indians. The dark shaded areas represent state in which the disease is prevalent.

challenge. We have seen hundreds of patients and each day continue finding new cases. For example, during the first 6 months of 1974 we saw 101 cases among the 7307 new patients examined in the Centro Dermatologico Federico Lleras Acosta of Bogota. Because of this high incidence of actinic prurigo in our country, the importance of the lesions as a cause of social disability, and the lack of any therapy of proven efficacy, a number of drugs have been tried in these patients on an empirical basis. It was on this basis that we tried the drug thalidomide, which we had used for several years in the treatment of erythema nodosum leprosum with great success and without side effects.

Our initial work (11) with this drug in the treatment of actinic prurigo was an uncontrolled trial with 34 patients. We used a dosage of 300 mg daily in adults and proportional doses in children, calculated on the basis of weight. This dosage was maintained until significant improvement had been observed and was then slowly reduced. Thirty-two of 34 patients showed considerable improvement, one patient showed

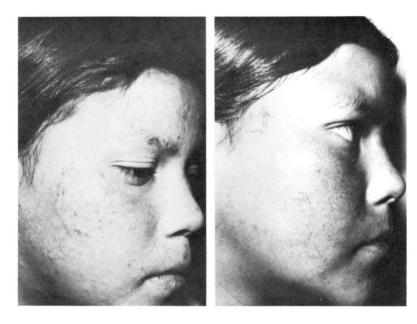

10 Response of actinic prurigo to thalidomide. Left: pretreatment. Right: posttreatment

slight improvement, and the remaining patient none. Figure 10 shows a typical clinical response. On the basis of our results with this uncontrolled study, we carried out a controlled, blind-randomized trial comparing thalidomide to three different cyclic imide derivatives of thalidomide (12). These latter compounds were treated as control drugs, in the absence of placebos which were not used. These three cyclic imides have a similar chemical structure to thalidomide, but, according to experiments with rats, do not have teratogenic action. The results of this study are summarized in Table I. Of 30 patients treated, 17 received thalidomide and 13 the other drugs. In 13 of the 17 patients who received thalidomide the results were excellent and in the remaining 4 the results were good. In the control group, which received the other cyclic imides, 3 of the 13 patients had excellent results, 3 good, and the remaining 7 no effect. Statistical evaluation of these results by Brant–Snedecor indicated a statistically significant superiority of thalidomide over the other drugs, in spite of the fact that the control drugs were

Table I. Randomized Trial of Thalidomode and Cyclic Imides

Drug	Response (%)			Total
	Excellent	Good	Poor	
Thalidomide	13 (76%)	4 (24%)	0	17
Cyclic imides	3 (23%)	3 (23%)	7 (54%)	13
Total	16	7	7	30

not inactive. Figure 11 shows the response to thalidomide therapy in two of the patients from the study. At present we are continuing to use thalidomide as the routine treatment for actinic prurigo and have had continuing favorable results.

It is of interest that in all of the cases treated the time necessary to obtain improvement was longer than that needed for the remission of symptoms in erythema nodosum leprosum. Table II shows the time required for both limited and marked improvement in both the uncontrolled and controlled trials. Despite considerable variation from patient to patient in the time required for clinical response, the average number of days required in the two studies were comparable (26 and 35 days for limited improvement and 49 and 52 days for marked improvement).

The asymptomatic period following the discontinuation of therapy was also variable (Table III). Some patients relapsed immediately on discontinuation of therapy, whereas others remained asymptomatic for more than 1 year.

DISCUSSION

On the basis of the clinical and epidemiological findings discussed, we believe that actinic prurigo should be separated from the group classified as chronic polymorphous light eruption. We also feel that the data here presented indicate that thalidomide is efficacious in the treatment of actinic prurigo. Although the mechanism of action of this drug is not clear, it could well be different from that proposed for its effect in erythema nodosum leprosum. The latter disease is a disorder of immune complexes whereas neither circulating nor tissue-fixed immunoglobulins have been described in actinic prurigo. Histopathologi-

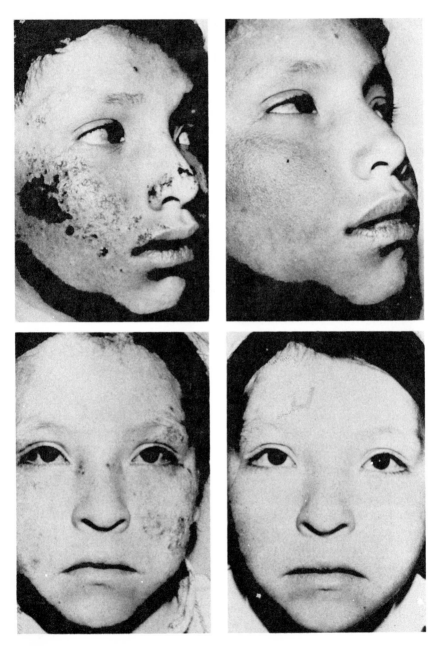

11 Response of patients with actinic prurigo to thalidomide therapy in a double blind study comparing thalidomide with other cyclic imides (see text for details).

Table II. Time Necessary for Improvement

Study	Average number of days (range)	
	Mild improvement	Marked improvement
Uncontrolled	26 (2-64)	49 (21-82)
Controlled	35 (14-62)	52 (27-85)

Table III. Time to Relapse in 40 Patients

Relapse	No. of patients
Immediate	9
<1 Month	2
1-6 Months	14
6-12 Months	8
>12 Months	7
	40

cally, the two diseases also differ in that the effector cells of the damage in erythema nodosum leprosum are polymorphonuclear leucocytes, which are thought to cause damage through the release of their lysosomal enzymes, whereas these cells are not seen in actinic prurigo, the infiltrate consisting of lymphocytes and histocytes. The two diseases also differ in the time course of their response to thalidomide, erythema nodosum leprosum responding in a matter of hours or days while the onset of action in actinic prurigo is a matter of weeks or even months.

In view of the differences in the pathogenesis of these two conditions and the different time courses of response to thalidomide, it is possible or even likely that this drug acts by different mechanisms in these two conditions. In erythema nodoum leprosum it has been postulated that thalidomide acts as a stabilizer of the lysosomal membranes of the polymorphonuclear leucocytes, therefore acting on the efferent limb of the immune response. It is obvious that this is an unlikely mechanism of action in the case of actinic prurigo since the predominant inflammatory cells are lymphocytes and histocytes. Because of the length

of time necessary for clinical response in this latter condition, Thalidomide could well be acting by inhibiting the afferent limb of an immune
response. Further investigation is required to determine the mechanism
of action in this disease and it is hoped that the knowledge so acquired
will enlighten us concerning the pathogenesis of actinic prurigo.

REFERENCES

1. G. Lopez Gonzalez, Prurigo solar. *Arch. Argent Dermatol.* IX, 301 (1961).
2. F. Londoño, Prurigo-eczema actinico. *Instantaneas Medicas* 49, 48 (1961).
3. H. Corrales, Dermatitis polimorfa por Luz. Su tratmiento con Trisora-len, *in* "Trabajo presentado al VII Congreso Ibero Latino Americano de Dermatologia." Caracas, 1971.
4. R.G. Hastings and M.J. Morales, Studies on the mechanism of Thalido-mides action (unpublished).
5. F. Cordero, personal communication, Guatemala, 1971.
6. R.R. Schenk, Controlled trials of Methoxalen in solar dermatitis of Chippewa Indians, *JAMA* 172, 1134 (1960).
7. M.A. Everett, W. Crochett and J.H. Lamb, Minor D: Lightsensitive eruptions in American Indians. *Arch. Dermatol.* 83, 243 (1961).
8. A.R. Birt, Photodermatitis in Indians of Manitoba. *Can. Med. Assn. J.* 98, 392 (1968).
9. F. Londoño, F. Muvdi, F. Gieraldo, L.A. Rueda, and A. Caputo, Familial actinic prurigo. *Dermatol. Ibero. Lat-AM.* 111, 61 (1968).
10. A.R. Birt and R.A. Davis, Photodermatitis in North American Indians: Familial actinic pruprigo. *Int. J. Dermatol.* 10, 107 (1971).
11. F. Londono, Thalidomide in the treatment of actinic prurigo. *Int. J. Dermatol.* 12, 326 (1973).
12. F. Londoño and M. Lopez, Tratamiento del Prurigo Actinico con Imidas Ciclicas. Unpublished

Recent Advances in Dermatopharmacology

15

Management of Pemphigus by the Intramuscular Administration of Gold Compounds

PHILLIP FROST
EDWARD C. GOMEZ

BACKGROUND

Pemphigus is a chronic, life-threatening bullous disease of mucocutaneous tissues in which characteristic antibodies are present in the serum and intercellular region of the epidermis of affected individuals.

Members of all races may develop the disease, but its incidence is higher in Jewish people and those of Mediterranean origin.

Pemphigus vegetans is a variant of pemphigus vulgaris in which hypertrophic lesions occur, particularly in intertrigenous areas. Pemphigus erythematosus is a minor form of pemphigus foliaceus, and fogo sevalgum is a South American epidemic form of pemphigus foliaceus. Generally, these variants have a less fulminant course than pemphigus vulgaris, although all can be fatal. Except for fogo sevalgum, which may occur in children, the onset is usually during adulthood. The various forms of pemphigus all have in common the presence of circulating antiepithelial antibodies (AEA).

Untreated, pemphigus vulgaris has a poor prognosis. It begins in the mouth in approximately 50% of affected patients and, eventually, almost all patients with pemphigus vulgaris develop blisters or erosions of the mouth or other mucous membranes. Before the advent of corticosteroids, the mortality rate from pemphigus vulgaris had been reported to be as high as 90% within a year of onset (1). Corticosteroid therapy has improved these frightful statistics, but since they must be administered chronically, and frequently in large doses, and since the disease commonly occurs in the elderly, eventual death or serious morbidity from the consequences of corticosteroids relegate this form of therapy to a less than satisfactory category (2,3).

The use of various antimetabolites such as methotrexate (4), cyclophosphamide (5), and azothioprine (6) has been described as useful in the management of pemphigus alone, in a few cases, or as an adjunct to corticosteroid therapy, in many cases. Recently, treating patients with pemphigus with gold sodium thiomalate or gold thioglucose either alone or after initial control of the disease with systemically administered corticosteroids has resulted in long-term remissions with no further therapy for periods as long as 34 months (7).

Becker and Obermayer (8) described quite casually the use of gold therapy for pemphigus: "some good results have been obtained by intravenous injections of gold compounds." The modern use of gold in medicine began with the observations of Koch that gold compounds were toxic *in vitro* for the tubercle bacillus. Later, Lande (9) and Forestier (10), noting the histologic similarities between tuberculosis and rheumatoid arthritis, treated patients with rheumatoid arthritis with gold compounds with favorable results. Although the use of gold to treat rheumatoid arthritis remained controversial for decades thereafter, carefully controlled studies eventually confirmed the findings of Lande and Forestier (11). It was because both rheumatoid arthritis and pemphigus have responded favorably to corticosteroids and immunosuppressive drugs and because characteristic humoral antibodies occur in both diseases that gold therapy was initially evaluated for the treatment of pemphigus (12).

CLINICAL STUDIES

Patient Selection

Pemphigus was diagnosed clinically and confirmed on histologic sections of biopsy specimens and by the presence of antiepithelial antibodies (AEA) in serum samples. Untreated patients or those receiving corticosteroids, either under control or with lesions, but with characteristic serum AEA demonstrable were included. Patients with pemphigus in whom gold therapy was contraindicated were excluded. All patients initially had a complete blood cell count, a urinalysis, a serum biochemical profile, an AEA titer determination, and a 24 hour urine sample collected for protein determination.

Gold Compounds

Initally, most of the patients were given gold sodium thiomalate (Myochrysine) as recommended in the package insert. Later, because of a shock-like reaction (nitritoid reaction) which may rarely occur with this compound but not with gold thioglucose (Solganol), and because both compounds appear to have equivalent efficacy in the treatment of pemphigus, gold thioglucose was used more. A test dose of 10 mg was given intramuscularly (I.M.), a week later 25 mg was administered I.M., followed by 50 mg I.M., at weekly intervals until the AEA titers fell significantly or until the patients' empirically determined need for corticosteroids decreased. At this point, the dose was either maintained at 50 mg/week, decreased to 50 mg on alternate weeks, or decreased to 25 mg a week until a cumulative dose of approximately 500 mg of the gold compound had been administered, at which point patients were given 25 mg or 50 mg every 2 to 4 weeks as part of a maintenance program. Attempts were periodically made to wean the patients from gold by decreasing the frequency or amount administered.

RESULTS

The results of the original studies in an initial group of 18 patients are summarized in Table I, and the results of a long term follow-up of 15 patients from this group are summarized in Table II. One group who had never received corticosteroids systemically for pemphigus consisted of three patients.

Case 1: A 71-year-old black lady who had only oral lesions when crysotherapy was begun developed blisters on her body during the course of gold therapy. When she had received a total of 610 mg of gold sodium thiomalate, AEA's were no longer detectable and her skin was clear. She received her gold over a period of 32 months and developed no new lesions during the 8 months following cessation of therapy. Mild persistent proteinuria developed after she had received 410 mg of gold sodium thiomalate.

Table I. Comparative Data in Two Methods of Therapy[a]

Patient no.	AEA titer		Gold sodium thiomalate dose, mg		Prednisone dose, mg	Complications	
	Before	After	Prednisone stopped[b]	Total to date		From prednisone	From gold sodium thiomalate
Patients who had never received corticosteroids systemically							
1	5,380	0	- - -	610	0	None	Nephrotic syndrome
2	80	0	- - -	485	0	None	None
3	160	0	- - -	885	0	None	None
Patients who have received corticosteroids systemically and who have responded to gold sodium thiomalate							
4	320	0	410	970	0	Diabetes, obesity, hypertension	Proteinuria
5	20	0	485	540	0	Cushingoid	Erythema nodosum
6	160	160	510	610	0	None	Dermatitis
7	2,560	20	485	835	0	Cushingoid, psychosis	None
8	40	0	285	385	0	Cushingoid	Agranulocytosis
9	320	0	660	910	10[c]	Hypoadrenalism	None
10	10	0	400	1,200	0	None	None
11	40	0	550	650	0	None	Dermatitis
12	1,240	0	310	995	0	None	None
13	320	0	290	390	0	None	None

164

Patients who have received corticosteroids systemically but who have not responded or responded poorly to gold sodium thiomalate

14	640	20	—	1,375	2.5	None	None
15	40	0	—	435	10	None	Dermatitis
16	10	0	- - -	450	30	None	None
17	160	0	- - -	1,110	10	None	None
18	320	80	- - -	795	60	None	None

[a]From Penneys et al, 1976.

[b]Total dose of gold sodium thiomalate at the time of cessation of systemically administered corticosteroids.

[c]After administration of 660 mg of gold sodium thiomalate, prednisone was discontinued. However, because of hypoadrenalism, low doses of systemically administered corticosteroid had to be readministered at a later date.

Tables I and II from the paper entitled "Management of Pemphigus with Gold Compounds" by Penneys, et al. (Archives of Dermatology, Vol. 112: 185-187, 1976).

165

Table II. Gold Dose and Length of Remission Without Therapy[a]

Case	Total gold received (mg)	Remission without therapy (mo)
1	1,520	8
2	1,685	...[b]
3	1,260	13
4	970	27
7	1,680	...[b]
9	780	34
10	895	...[b]
11	1,025	16
12	1,145	25
13	1,210	...[b]
14	2,825	...[b]
15	450	28
16	925	20
17	2,275	...[b]
18	1,480	...[b]

[a]From Penneys et al, 1976.
[b]... Receiving gold injections.

Case 2: A 78-year-old white man received 1685 mg of gold compound over a 3-year period. His AEA titer became undetectable and his skin lesions cleared by the time he had received 310 mg of gold compound, but cessation of therapy on sevaral occasions resulted in blister formation.

Case 3: A 52-year-old white woman with a 2 year history of oral and vaginal erosions developed no further lesions and had an undetectable AEA titer by the time she had received 610 mg of gold sodium thiomalate. She was maintained free of lesions on 25 mg of gold thiomalate bimonthly and remained free of lesions for 13 months following complete cessation of therapy except for a rare oral erosion which healed spontaneously.

A second group of patients initially received corticosteroids and then responded to gold therapy.

Case 4: A 60-year-old had originally required 20 mg of prednisone daily to keep free of oral lesions. After receiving 310 mg of gold sodium thiomalate, her AEA's were undetectable, her steroids were stopped, and she was kept free of lesions with 25 mg of gold compound every 2 or 3 weeks for 18 months. All therapy was then discontinued and she remained lesion-free for 27 months. Mild proteinuria led to temporary cessation of gold therapy which was then restarted without incident after her urine became free of protein.

Case 5: A 43-year-old white woman who still had numerous skin lesions and an AEA titer of 20 dilutions while taking 20 mg of prednisone daily cleared completely and had undetectable AEA on gold therapy. Prednisone therapy was discontinued but when she had received a total of 45 mg of gold compound, she developed eosinophilia, albuminuria, and a pityriasis rosea-like skin eruption. Gold therapy was stopped and resumed after these findings cleared, but the patient developed erythema nodosum requiring discontinuation of gold therapy (13).

Case 6: A 34-year-old white woman who still had numerous skin lesions after treatment with prednisone and methotrexate for 22 months was started on gold therapy. After receiving a total dose of 235 mg of gold compounds, lesions were no longer present. After receiving 360 mg of gold compound, she developed dermatitis and eosinophilia, both of which resolved 1 week after withholding gold therapy. Gold was then started again without incident and when she had received 510 mg of gold compound, prednisone was stopped with no further development of skin lesions, although her AEA titer remained at 100 dilutions. She was subsequently lost to follow-up.

Case 7: A 59-year-old man with severe skin lesions and an AEA titer of 2560 was placed on chrysotherapy and systemic prednisone. Corticosteroids were discontinued when his skin was clear, at which time he had received 485 mg of gold compound. He was then kept free of blisters for over 2 years with 25 mg of gold compound a month as his only form of therapy.

Case 8: A 58-year-old white man with pemphigus for 5 years had required up to 350 mg of orally administered prednisone daily for control. At the beginning of gold therapy, his AEA titer was 80 dilutions and severe oral cavity and facial erosions were present despite daily treatment with 350 mg of prednisone. When his total dose of gold sodium thiomalate was 285 mg, he developed agranulocytosis and was admitted to the hospital. He had also been taking chlorpropamide (Diabinese) and amitriptyline hydrochloride (Elavil). The patient died suddenly of respiratory arrest in the hospital after recovering from the agranulocytosis. An autopsy was not performed.

Case 9: An 80-year-old woman with severe pemphigus recalcitrant to systemic prednisone therapy was given chrysotherapy, in addition to the prednisone, until her skin was completely clear. Prednisone was continued at a dose of 10 mg daily to avoid hypoadrenalism but this was eventually discontinued. Gold therapy was also discontinued after the patient had received a total dose of 780 mg of gold compound and she remained in remission for the following 34 months.

Case 10: A 73-year-old man was treated for a severe exacerbation of pemphigus with prednisone and gold sodium thiomalate. Prednisone was discontinued after the patient was free of lesions, had undetectable AEA's, and had received a total of 400 mg of gold compound. He has remained free of lesions on maintenance gold therapy. No attempts have been made to discontinue the gold therapy.

Case 11: A 71-year-old man with only erosions of the mouth was treated with orally administered triamcinolone diacetate or prednisone and gold sodium thiomalate. His mouth lesions cleared and he developed gold dermatitis when the corticosteroids were discontinued, at which time he had received 575 mg of gold compound. Gold therapy was interrupted and his dermatitis cleared within a month. He later developed another blister on his lip which cleared after an additional 450 mg of gold compound were administered. He remained free of lesions for 36 months following cessation of all therapy.

Case 12: A 23-year-old woman who developed pemphigus at age 19 was managed initially with systemically given corticosteroids and then with chrysotherapy. After receiving maintenance chrysotherapy for 1 year, all medications were discontinued. No lesions developed during the subsequent 25 months.

Case 13: A 67-year-old woman had an AEA titer of 320 dilutions when chrysotherapy was begun. After 290 mg of gold compound were administered, the prednisone was stopped, at which point her AEA titer was 0. She has required 25 mg of gold compound every second or fourth week, since cessation of gold therapy has resulted in blister formation.

A third group of patients did not initially respond to gold therapy; some did eventually.

Case 14: A 55-year-old man with oral lesions of pemphigus which required large doses of prednisone to control was treated with gold sodium thiomalate. After receiving a total of 2825 mg of gold compound, he still requires 5 mg of prednisone daily and still develops an occasional oral erosion.

Case 15: A 78-year-old man died on October 1, 1974 of causes unrelated to pemphigus or its treatment. His last gold injection was in August 1972. For 28 months prior to his death, he took 5 mg of prednisone daily and exhibited no signs of active pemphigus.

Case 16: A 71-year-old woman still required 60 mg of prednisone on alternate days to control her pemphigus after receiving 450 mg of gold compound. After receiving a total of 925 mg of gold compound, however, she went into remission except for an occasional rapidly resolving oral erosion with no therapy at all for over 20 months.

Case 17: Pemphigus in a 68-year-old man was poorly controlled with systemic corticosteroid therapy. Chrysotherapy begun in 1971 gradually reduced the steroid requirement. For the last 30 months, he has been on a maintenance schedule. Attempts at cessation of chrysotherapy resulted in blister formation. Occasional blisters have developed on gold therapy, necessitating short courses of systemically administered corticosteroids.

Case 18: A 74-year-old man had severe pemphigus foliaceous, requiring a minimum of 75 mg of prednisone daily to control the eruption. Two courses of chrysotherapy were given. The first course of 795 mg was entirely without benefit. During the ensuing year, his disease was managed with high doses of prednisone (75–100 mg daily) or with a parentarally administered, experimental, long acting, synthetic corticotropin compound (BA41795, Ciba). The corticotropin preparation controlled the eruption completely, but the side effects of the drug were debilitating. Chrysotherapy consisting of 50 mg weekly was reinstituted in March, 1974. His response was equivocal,

Table III. Side Effects

Dermatitis and stomatitis (most common)
  pruritis
  morbiliform eruption
  exfoliative dermatitis
  lichen planus like eruption
  pustular dermatitis
  petechial or purpuric eruption
  erythema nodosum
  pityriasis rosea like eruption
  glossitis, gingivitis, stomatitis

Conjunctivitis, iritis, corneal ulcer

Eosinophilia, leukopenia, agranulocytosis, anemia,
  thrombocytopenia, aplastic anemia

Blurring of vision, meningitis, polyneuritis

Albuminuria, hematuria, nephrosis

"Nitritoid" reactions

Lymphadenitis

Non-productive cough, "gold bronchitis"

Gastrointestinal disturbances
  nausea, vomiting
  diarrhea
  abdominal pain
  hepatitis, jaundice

---

allowing a reduction in prednisone dosage from 75 mg daily to 35 mg daily. An intensive course of chrysotherapy is now being given to this patient.

GOLD TOXICITY

The toxic side effects of gold compounds are listed in Table III. Skin eruptions and stomatitis are the most common reactions. They are usually not severe and may not reoccur if gold therapy is cautiously resumed after interrupting gold therapy long enough for the eruptions to subside. Exfoliative dermatitis, erythema nosodum, and purpuric

Table IV. Contraindications to Gold Therapy[a]

Absolute
disseminated lupus erythematosus
pregnancy
Relative (may be used, but with extreme caution)
cardiac, renal, hepatic disease
marked hypertension
severe diabetes mellitus
chronic skin disorders
ulcerative colitis
severe anemia
history of agranulocytosis, purpura, hemorrhagic
tendancy, other blood cyscrasias

[a]Package insert for Myochrysine (gold sodium thiomalate) Merck and Co., Inc.

eruptions are more serious, of course, and, in most cases, would preclude futher therapy with gold compounds. Eosinophilia frequently occurs and may precede toxic skin reactions.

Of the 18 patients with pemphigus treated with gold in this series, four developed a skin reaction. One (Case 5), developed erythema nodosum, which required cessation of gold therapy.

Two patients developed proteinuria which did not require cessation of gold therapy. Mild albuminuria may occur in many patients but is not necessarily a contraindication to continued chrysotherapy. Such patients should, however, be carefully watched. If albuminuria becomes more pronounced or persistent, the dose should be reduced or chrysotherapy should be discontinued temporarily. Treatment should be stopped if albuminuria is severe.

One patient (Case 8) developed agranulocytosis which was resolving when he died of unrelated causes. The mechanism of gold toxicity in hematopoietic as well as other tissues is not known. The occurrence of gold toxicity is not particularly related to gold levels in any tissue, although toxicity does not usually occur before the cumulative dose of gold administered is in the therapeutic range (300–500 mg) (13).

The contraindications to gold therapy listed in Table IV are clearly related to the possible toxic effects of gold listed in Table III. Most contraindications are relative, indicating that, with extreme care, gold may be administered.

PHARMACOLOGY

Gold is absorbed within 1 hour after intramuscular injection of gold sodium thiomalate or gold thioglucose. With increasing doses at weekly intervals, the gold plasma concentration increases in stepwise fashion. Between injections, the daily plasma levels may fluctuate somewhat, but generally they remain constant or decrease slightly until the next injection. Plasma gold levels are higher after large doses, but these levels are not directly related to the weekly gold intake.

Gold is eliminated mainly by the kidneys, although a small amount appears in the feces. On weekly doses of 50 mg of gold (100 mg of gold compound) about 1 mg is excreted daily. Thus, more than 80% of a dose is present in the body after 1 week, the usual interval between injections. As increased amounts of gold are given, the urinary excretion increases, but not proportionately. Thus, the percentage of retained gold increases with increasing dosage. Following completion of a course, gold may appear in the plasma and urine for 6 to 12 months, when large doses have been given, and for a correspondingly shorter period, with smaller doses.

DISCUSSION

The simple thrust of this review is that gold therapy for pemphigus appears to offer hope for long term remission without further therapy of any kind for a significant percentage of patients treated (Table II). These results are above and beyond those achieved with other forms of therapy and the associated toxicity of gold therapy appears to be of significantly lesser magnitude than that associated with chronic corticosteroid therapy.

The mechanism of action of gold in the treatment of pemphigus is known, as is the case with rheumatoid arthritis. Neither antibody production, interaction of antibody and antigen, or other immunologic parameters have been demonstrated to be affected by chrysotherapy.

REFERENCES

1. S. Gellis and F.A. Glass, Pemphigus: A survey of 170 patients admitted to Bellevue Hospital from 1911 to 1941. *Arch. Dermatol. Syph.* 44, 321–336 (1941).

2. J.G. Ryan, Pemphigus: A 20-year survey of experience with 70 cases. *Arch. Dermatol.* 104, 14–20 (1971).
3. F.R. Rosenberg, S. Sanders, and C.T. Nelson, Pemphigus: A 20-year review of 107 patients treated with corticosteroids. *Arch. Dermatol.* 112, 962–970 (1976).
4. W.F. Lever, Methotrexate and Prednisone in pemphigus vulgaris: Therapeutic results obtained in 36 patients between 1961 and 1970. *Arch. Dermatol.* 106, 491–497 (1972).
5. E.M. McKelvey and J. Hasegawa, Cyclophosphamide and Pemphigus Vulgaris. *Arch Dermatol.* 103, 198–200 (1971).
6. H.H. Roenigk and S. Deodhar, Pemphigus treatment with azathioprine: Clinical and immunologic correlation. *Arch. Dermatol.* 107, 353–357 (1973).
7. N.S. Penneys, W.H. Eaglstein, and P. Frost, Management of pemphigus with gold compounds: A long-term follow-up report. *Arch. Dematol.* 112, 185–187 (1976).
8. S.W. Becker and M.E. Obermayer, "Modern Dermatology and Syphilology, p. 139. J B Lippincott, Co, Philadelphia, 1947.
9. K. Lande, *Munchen med. Wochschr.* 74, 1132 (1927).
10. J. Forestier, *Bull. mem. Soc. med. hop. Paris* 53, 329 (1929).
11. Cooperating Clinics Committee of the American Rheumatism Association, A controlled trial of gold salt therapy in rheumatoid arthritis. *Arthritis Rheum.* 16, 353–358 (1973).
12. N.S. Penneys, W.H. Eaglstein, A. Indgin, and P. Frost, Gold sodium thiomalate treatment of pemphigus. *Arch. Dermatol.* 108, 55–60 (1973).
13. R.L. Stone, A. Claflin, and N.S. Penneys, Erythema nodosum following gold therapy. *Arch. Dermatol.* 107, 602–604 (1973).
14. N.L. Gottlieb, P.M. Smith, N.S. Penneys et al., Gold concentrations in hair, nail, and skin during chrysotherapy. *Arthritis Rheum.* 17, 56–62 (1974).

16

Mycophenolic Acid for Psoriasis

E. LINN JONES

Mycophenolic acid is a weakly acidic antibiotic produced by fermentation of *Penicillium stoloniferum*. It is a white, odorless, bitter crystalline substance. The structural formula is shown in Fig. 1. Mycophenolic acid is one of the oldest known antibiotics. It has limited antibacterial and antifungal action, but these have no apparent clinical utility (1,2).

In screens for prospective antitumor drugs, mycophenolic acid was found to retard the growth of several solid murine tumors but was inactive against murine leukemias (3–5). Beginning in 1969, clinical trials in cancer patients were initiated in the United States and England. To date, the drug has not proven useful as a antitumor agent for man, however, these clinical trials indicated that the compound had a low degree of toxicity (6–8).

Because of the effectiveness of certain other antitumor drugs in psoriasis, mycophenolic acid was subjected to trials in that disease by both the oral and topical route in 1971. When mycophenolic acid was applied to uninvolved skin of psoriasis patients under occlusive dressings it produced, after 7 to 10 days, a primary irritation reaction characterized

$$HO_2C \: CH_2CH_2\underset{\underset{CH_3}{|}}{C}=CHCH_2$$

1   Structural formula of mycophenolic acid.

by redness, edema, and a spongiotic dermatitis with erosion. The irritation was related to concentration. Application in a similar manner to involved skin in psoriasis patients did not produce irritation, but did not improve lesions to any significant degree at the dose level employed (9). In contrast, the oral route of administration appears to be effective when adequate doses are given (10).

An extensive study of related compounds indicated that for anticancer activity the phenolic group of the molecule must be present in an unblocked state or susceptible to hydrolysis (11). When the phenolic group is esterified to yield mycophenolic acid glucuronide, the resulting compound is inactive, presumably due to an inability to penetrate cell membranes (12).

Man and rabbit are among the more rapid esterifiers of mycophenolic acid. This capability presumably accounts for their ability to tolerate higher doses than other animals, such as the mouse and rat (13).

PHARMACODYNAMICS

The epidermal cells in the lesions of psoriasis are known to have a cell cycle that is much more rapid than normal. Mycophenolic acid is thought to slow this excessive growth rate by entering the epidermal

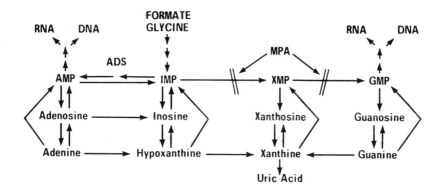

2   Site of metabolic blockade produced by mycophenolic acid (MPA).

cells and interfering with the synthesis of purine precursors of RNA and DNA (11).

To date, however, we have no direct evidence that the drug actually enters the epidermal cell or has a direct action at that location. Attempts to detect the drug in the shed scales of psoriatic epidermis have not been successful (14). Addition of mycophenolic acid to a tissue culture medium containing freshly excised human skin did not reduce thymidine incorporation in epidermal cells during a 2-hour incubation (15). The lack of significant antipsoriatic effect on topical application also raises doubts concerning a direct action in epidermal cells.

Psoriatic patients have been shown to have certain abnormalities in their immune processes (16–18). It is possible that mycophenolic acid has an indirect beneficial effect on the skin through an alteration in the immune mechanisms. Such a mechanism would help to explain the beneficial effects that have been observed in psoriatic arthritis and in experimental animal arthritis (19,20).

Mycophenolic acid interferes with two enzymes, namely, inosine monophosphate dehydrogenase which converts inosine monophosphate to xanthosine monophosphate (21), and guanosine monophosphate synthetase which converts xanthosine monophosphate to guanosine monophosphate (22). Figure 2 illustrates the sites of this metabolic blockade. The biologic effects of such a blockade can be overcome by addition of guanosine to tissue culture media. Mycophenolic acid is thought to bind to both enzymes at sites other than the sites which bind the enzyme substrates, since the bindings of the compounds are not competitive (21).

Several biochemical effects of the drug have been observed. In a group of patients with psoriasis followed over an 8-week period, a 25% reduction in IgG was observed. This degree of reduction was statistically significant (p less than 0.05) (23). The drug produces a compensatory elevation of inosine monophosphate dehydrogenase in circulating red blood cells (24). Reduction of blood uric acid occurs in psoriasis patients (10).

PHARMACOKINETICS

After oral administration mycophenolic acid appears to be absorbed rapidly and completely. In a study utilizing a single 1200 mg oral dose, less than 1% of the drug was recovered in the feces. The bulk of the drug was recovered in the urine in the form of either mycophenolic acid glucuronide or free mycophenolic acid (25). When animals were fed ^{14}C–labeled drug, no $^{14}CO_2$ was detected in the expired air, indicating that mycophenolic acid is not metabolically degraded (11).

When an oral dose of 1200 mg was given without food to six male volunteers in a fasting state, a peak blood level of 21 mcg/ml (range 18–48) was achieved at 1 hour following ingestion. By 8 hours this mean had declined to 2.8 mcg/ml. Mycophenolic acid glucuronide reached a mean peak level of 44 mcg/ml (range 31–69) at 3 hours after ingestion. By 8 hours this mean had declined to 22 mcg/ml. These data illustrate the relatively short half-life of mycophenolic acid as it is rapidly transformed into the glucuronide. Forthy-eight-hour urine collections following a 1200 mg dose recovered 82% of the administered doses. The actual excretion was probably higher than this, since creatinine analysis provided evidence of some incomplete urine collections in the study. In each instance, less than 3% of the drug recovered in the urine was excreted as the free mycophenolic acid. The bulk of the drug was present as the glucuronide (25).

Although individuals show considerable variation in response of their psoriasis to the drug, the biochemical or genetic basis for this variation is unknown.

CINICAL PHARMACOLOGY

Initial clinical trials involved cancer patients treated with the water-soluble salt, sodium mycophenolate, by intramuscular or intravenous routes. In tolerance studies several patients received doses equivalent to 4–8 gm of mycophenolic acid in the form of a 24-hour continuous I.V. drip. One patient received 10 gm/day for 4 consecutive days. A plasma level of 232 mcg/ml was achieved, with almost all of the drug in the glucuronide form. Later, this patient received the equivalent of 14 gm of mycophenolic acid per day and achieved a blood level of 300 mcg/ml of plasma, almost all as glucuronide (26).

A pilot study was conducted with oral mycophenolic acid in psoriasis patients between 1971 and 1973. In a group of 29 patients the maximum tolerated dose was found to range from 2400 to 4800 mg/day, or 30 to 96 mg/Kg ideal weight/day. The characteristic dose-limiting side-effects were found to be soft or frequent bowel movements, diarrhea, nausea, and anorexia. The drug produced a reduction in disease elements such as redness, scaling, and thickening of psoriatic plaques, sensations of pain, burning and itching arising in the skin, fissuring of psoriatic lesions, and the percent of body surface area involved with redness and scaling. The full effect of the drug required a median time of 8 weeks. with a range of 5–14 weeks. This onset time is thought to be longer than that of methotrexate in psoriasis. When mycophenolic acid was discontinued, relapses occurred with a median time of 4 weeks (range 3–8). Fifteen of the 29 patients achieved almost complete or complete clearing of their lesions (10).

The efficacy of mycophenolic acid in psoriasis has been confirmed by five independent placebo-controlled, double-blind parallel studies. The results of one of these are shown in Fig. 3.

DOSAGE

A typical dosage regimen is shown below

Week	Dosage
1	800 mg q 8 hours
2	1200 mg q 8 hours
3–16	1600 mg q 8 hours

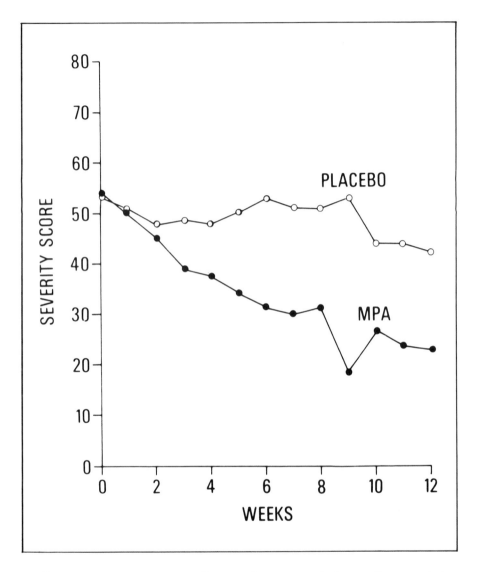

3   Decrease in mean psoriasis severity score during treatment with mycophenolic acid or placebo.

An alternate regimen which is expected to produce a lower risk of adverse reaction, is as follows

Week	
1 and 2	800 mg q 12 hours with food
3 and 4	1200 mg q 12 hours with food
5–16	1600 mg q 12 hours with food

If adverse reactions are encountered, interrupt the treatment for 2 days, then resume the same or a lower dose. Postpone increases unless the current dose is well tolerated.

In general, dosage should start with approximately 30 mg/Kg/day and increase depending upon adverse reactions and response to 96 mg/Kg/day in divided doses every 8 or 12 hours. Dosage for obese patients should be based on their ideal weights, rather than their actual weights. The average maintenance dose for psoriasis patients is approximately 60 mg/Kg ideal weight/day.

Since the drug might interfere with the processes involved in immune responses, inflammation, wound healing, and repair, it is good practice to interrupt the drug for infections, wounds, fractures. surgery, infarctions, thrombosis, and vaccinations.

When patients are on extended trips and vacations and unable to meet laboratory monitoring schedules, the drug should be discontinued.

When gastrointestinal reactions limit the dosage, switching from an 8-hour dose interval to a 12- or 24-hour dose interval may provide a better ratio of response to adverse effects.

Certain patients appear to be "nonresponders," even when doses as high as 100 mg/Kg/day can be tolerated. If such a dose does not give satisfactory clearing after 16 weeks, discontinuation of the medicine should be considered. On the other hand, some patients appear to be "slow responders" and may require up to 12 months to achieve their full response to the drug. The basis for this variation in response is unknown.

PRECAUTIONS IN USING THE DRUG

Before treatment the following laboratory tests are advised:

Hematology
  WBC and differential
  RBC or hematocrit
  Hemoglobin
  Platelet count

Renal studies
  Urinalysis
  BUN
Liver function
  Routine liver function tests such as SGOTransaminase
  LDH
  Alkaline phosphatase
  BSP (optional)

A BSP might be considered if abnormalities are seen in the other liver function tests or the patient is a heavy drinker. In the case of younger male patients who might be concerned about the effect on spermatogenesis, a baseline pretreatment semen analysis may be obtained, along with a second analysis after 12 to 16 weeks of treatment.

For the safety of the patient, the following schedule of laboratory tests is recommended: WBC, RBC, and platelets—before treatment and after 1, 2, 4, 6, 8, 12, and 16 weeks. Then repeat every 4 or 8 weeks during treatment. Blood chemistry and Urinalysis—before treatment and after 12 weeks. Renal studies and liver studies should be repeated every 6 months during treatment.

Since influenza can cause a transient neutropenia, patients should be advised to discontinue the drug if symptoms of influenza should arise, and not resume the drug until the neutrophil count has been checked and found to have returned to normal.

Patients with urinary tract symptoms occurring before or during treatment should have urine cultures and sensitivity studies. Patients with a history of gastric or duodenal ulcer may need an ulcer regimen while using mycophenolic acid. The safety of the drug has not been studied in patients with ulcerative colitis or irritable bowel syndrome.

The safety and effectiveness of the drug has not been studied in children under 12.

ADVERSE REACTIONS AND THEIR MANAGEMENT

In the early weeks of treatment, the patient may experience nausea, reduced appetite, and even vomiting. Nausea can be reduced by advising the patient to take a small amount of food with the drug. The morning and afternoon doses are more likely to produce nausea than the bedtime dose. Frequently nausea can be controlled by redistributing the daily dose in an unequal manner, thereby reducing the dose at the time at which nausea is more frequently encountered. Obese patients, unfortunately, seldom notice a reduction in appetite.

Later in the course of treatment, typically 3 to 6 weeks, patients may encounter abdominal cramps, distention, bloating. passage of gas, soft or more frequent bowel movements, diarrhea, and tenderness in the mouth or rectum. If these effects are minor and easily tolerated, it may not be necessary to reduce or interrupt the dosage. When they are more serious the drug can be interrupted for 48 hours and then resumed at the same or a lower dose. Some investigators have found that the use of Lomotil® or the bulk producing laxative, Konsyl®, helps to control the hypermotility of the bowel.

Signs of bladder irritation, such as frequent or urgent urination or burning during or after urination, have been observed, especially among women. Such symptoms may arise from a latent urinary tract infection or may be the result of a direct irritating action of the drug itself.

Central nervous system effects include weakness or fatigue, insomnia, lightheadedness, or even fainting. When insomnia, weakness, or fatigue occur, the adverse reactions seem to be chronic and are relieved only by interrupting the drug or reducing the dosage. For certain patients these are the dose-limiting adverse reactions. Some investigators have found the hypnotic drug, Dalmane®, useful in controlling the insomnia.

Semen analyses have revealed that a transient, but often marked, decline in sperm count may occur in the first 2–6 weeks of treatment, followed by a return toward pretreatment levels. This response is seen primarily in patients that are hypospermic or at the lower limit of normality prior to treatment.

Long-term safety studies indicate that uninterrupted treatment may be associated with an increased risk of herpes zoster. To date, such zoster episodes have been typical in severity and duration.

The adverse reactions produced by the drug are proportional to the daily dose. The drug is better tolerated when taken with a 12- or 24-hour-dose interval than with an 8-hour-dose interval, but it may be less effective as the dose interval is extended.

Other drugs which tend to cause GI irritation, such as erythromycin or iron, may add to the bowel irritability problem of mycophenolic acid patients. No other drug interactions have been observed to date. Special care might be advisable when patients are under treatment with digitoxin, anticoagulants, or other drugs with a critical dosage.

Free mycophenolic acid fluoresces in blood and urine. It may interfere with laboratory tests based on fluorescence.

CONCLUSION

Mycophenolic acid offers the potential of almost complete clearing or definite improvement in most patients with psoriasis.

REFERENCES

1. E.P. Abraham, The effect of mycophenolic acid on the growth of *Staphylococcus aureus* in heart broth. *Biochem. J.* 39, 398–408 (1945).
2. H.W. Florey, K. Gilliver, M.A. Jennings, and A.G. Sanders. Mycophenolic acid, an antibiotic from *Penicillium brevi-compactum* Dierckx. *Lancet* 1, 46–49 (1946).
3. R.H. Williams, D.H. Lively, D.E. Delong, J.C. Cline, M.J. Sweeney, G.A. Poore, and S.H. Larsen, Mycophenolic acid. Antiviral and antitumor properties. *J. Antibiot. (Tokyo)* 21, 463–464 (1968).
4. M.J. Sweeney, J.C. Cline, and R.H. Williams, Antitumor and antiviral activities of mycophenolic acid (abstr). *Proc. Am. Assoc. Cancer Res* 10, 90 (1969).
5. M.J. Sweeney, K. Gerzon, P.N. Harris, R.E. Holmes, G.A. Poore, and R.H. Williams, Experimental antitumor activity and preclinical toxicology of mycophenolic acid. *Cancer Res.* 32, 1795–1802 (1972).
6. T.B. Brewin, M.P. Cole, C.T.A. Jones, D.S. Platt, and I.D.H. Todd, Mycophenolic acid (NSC–129185), Preliminary clinical trials. *Cancer Chemother. Rep. Part 1*, 56, 83–87 (1972).
7. S. Knudtzon, N.I. Nissen, Clinical trial with mycophenolic acid (NSC–129185), a new antitumor agent. *Cancer Chemother. Rep. Part 1* 56, 221–227 (1972).
8. J. Lintrup, P. Hyltoft-Peterson, S. Kundtzon, and N.I. Nissen, Metabolic studies in man with mycophenolic acid (NSC–129185), a new antitumor agent. *Cancer Chemother. Rep. Part 1* 56, 229–235 (1972).
9. E.L. Jones, Unpublished observations.
10. E.L. Jones, W.W. Epinette, V.C. Hackney, L. Menendez, and P. Frost, Treatment of psoriasis with oral mycophenolic acid. *J. Invest. Dermatol.* 65, 537–542 (1975).
11. M.J. Sweeney, unpublished observations.
12. M.J. Sweeney, D.H. Hoffman, and M.A. Esterman, Metabolism and biochemistry of mycophenolic acid. *Cancer Res.* 32, 1803–1809 (1972).
13. E. Adams, G. Todd, and W. Gibson, Long term toxicity study of mycophenolic acid in rabbits. *Toxicol and Applied Pharmacol.* 34, 509–512 (1975).
14. R.L. Wolen, unpublished observations.
15. R. Fleischmajer, unpublished observations.

16. S. Sandnerr, J. Foussere, and A. Basset, 2,4-Dinitrochlorobenzene sensitization of psoriatic patients. *Contact Dermatitis* 1, 184–186 (1975).
17. W.L. Epstein, Immunologic factors in psoriasis. *Psoriasis, Proc. Int. Symp. Stanford University, 1971* (E.M. Farber and A.J. Cox eds.), Stanford University Press, Stanford, California, 1971.
18. J. Clot, E. Charmasson, H. Massip, J.J. Guilhou, J. Meynadier, Deficit des T-lymphocytes das le psoriasis. *Nouvelle Presse Medicale* 4, 2039–2040 (1975).
19. E.L. Jones, Treatment of arthritis with mycophenolic acid and derivatives, U.S. Patent No. 3,880,995 (1975).
20. K.A. Martlage, unpublished observations.
21. T.J. Franklin and J.M. Cook, The inhibition of nucleic acid synthesis by mycophenolic acid. *Biochem. J.* 113, 515–524 (1969).
22. M.J. Sweeney, unpublished observations.
23. B. Petersen and E.L. Jones, unpublished observations.
24. E.W. Holmes, W.H. Turner, and J.P. Tindall, Increased inosinic acid dehydrogenase activity in patients receiving mycophenolic acid for psoriasis (abstr). *Clin. Res.* 23, 23A (1975).
25. C. Gruber, A. Rubin, P. Warrick and B.E. Rodda, unpublished observations.
26. R.W. Dyke, unpublished observations.

Recent Advances in Dermatopharmacology

17

8-Methoxypsoralen and Ultraviolet Light for Psoriasis

JOHN A. PARRISH

Oral ingestion of 8-methoxypsoralen (8-MOP, methoxsalen) and subsequent exposure to longwave ultraviolet light (320–400 nm, UV-A) leads to erythema and pigmentation of normal human skin. Multiple drug and light exposures lead to improvement and then to complete clearing of psoriasis vulgaris. The combination of drug and light to bring about a beneficial effect has been termed photochemotherapy.

THE DRUG

Psoralens are furocoumarins, some of which can absorb energy from ultraviolet radiation and thereby induce photochemical reactions in the skin. These tricyclic compounds can be synthesized by adding a furan ring to a suitably substituted coumarin (benz-α-pyrone or 1,2-benzopyrine) derivative (1). In addition, 28 psoralens are found in plants or can be isolated from microorganisms (2). Two psoralens are commercially available in the United States; 4, 5', 8-trimethylpsoralen (TMP) is synthesized, and methoxsalen (8-MOP, 8-methoxypsoralen,

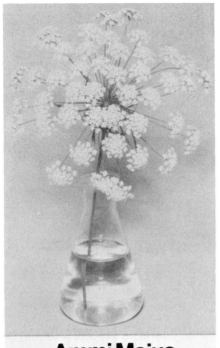

OCH3

8-methoxypsoralen (8-MOP)

Ammi Majus

1   *Ammi Majus L.,* is the source of 8-methoxypsoralen.

xanthotoxin) is obtained from *Ammi majus L.,* a plant found in the Nile Valley (Fig. 1).

Although the absorption spectra for 8-MOP and TMP lies between 210 and 330 nm (1) the action spectrum for photosensitization and photochemical changes is wavelengths longer than 320 nm. The drug can photosensitize the skin after oral or topical administration.

THE LIGHT

Electromagnetic energy from the sun or various artificial sources forms a continuum of electrostatic and magnetic force which has the properties of waves and also has the properties of a stream of particles.

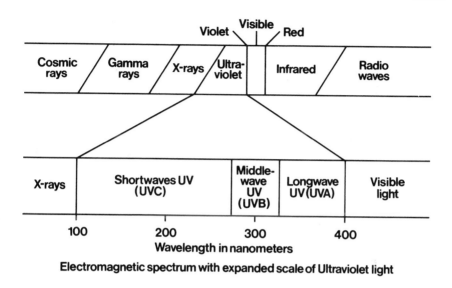

Electromagnetic spectrum with expanded scale of Ultraviolet light

2

The electromagnetic spectrum.

While any separation or catagorization of this continuum of energies is arbitrary and artificial, convention has given names to various portions of the electromagnetic spectrum depending on which atoms, molecules, or human receptors absorb or react with specific energy or photons. Because the electromagnetic forces move through a vacuum at the speed of light, there is an inverse relationship between wavelength and energy.

Figure 2 illustrates some of the names used to describe the portions of the ultraviolet spectrum. UV-B is the sunburn spectrum. Photons in this waveband region are very efficient in inducing erythema and pigmentation, and by cumulative processes probably cause skin cancer, actinic keratosis, aging, and wrinkling. UV-A is of longer wavelength, lower frequency, and less energy than UV-B. It is 1000 times less efficient at causing erythema and has been ignored for decades by cutaneous physiologists as biologically inactive.

Four important facts about UV-A have recently been called to the awareness of the dermatopharmacologist and dermatologist:

(1) UV-A can cause erythema. Newly developed light sources deliver enough energy to make UV-A light testing quantitative and practical. Sunscreens designed to scatter or absorb UV-B are so efficient that unpigmented persons can remain in the sun long enough to receive UV-A erythema. The erythemogenesis of UV-A can add to or augment sunburn erythema.

(2) The UV-A content of the sun is 10 to 100 or more times that of UV-B depending on season or time of day.

(3) UV-A penetrates deeper into the skin than do the shorter wavelength of higher frequency and more energetic photons; the latter are more easily scattered and more readily absorbed by proteins and DNA.

(4) Certain chemicals absorb UV-A and induce biologic alterations in living cells. The most photoactive of these compounds are the psoralens.

THE REACTIONS ON NORMAL SKIN

PUVA (psoralen and subsequent exposure to UV-A) causes an erythema reaction which has the appearance of sunburn but differs from normal sunburn in several ways. PUVA redness involves larger and deeper vessels than does sunburn and may have a violaceous hue. The PUVA erythema reaction may not be impressive at 12 to 24 hours after UV exposure, when sunburn usually is maximized, but instead does not reach its peak until 48 hours or later. As little as 2 or 3 times that UV-A dose which causes minimal redness may lead to pain, edema, and blistering. Because of these properties, daily PUVA exposures carry risk of cumulative erythema reactions which may lead to severe burns.

PUVA erythema is followed by true melanogenesis. Light and electron microscopic studies suggest that the melanocyte is stimulated and altered immediately but tanning is not noticeable until several days after exposure and maximizes at about 5–7 days. Although tanning response is variable and limited by a person's genetic ability to pigment, one or two erythemogenic PUVA exposures can maximally stimulate true melanogenesis. There is some evidence that topical psoralens and UV-A may in fact alter the average melanosome size and thereby influence the packaging or grouping of melanosomes within the keratinocytes (3).

Repeated PUVA exposures may lead to gradual thickening of the stratum corneum. Hundreds of phototoxic reactions over many years may cause hyperkeratosis and aged appearance of unprotected amelanotic (vitiligo) skin.

POSSIBLE MECHANISMS

In the presence of UV-A, psoralens undergo photoexcitation and transition of the photoexcited singlet state psoralen molecule to its triplet state. This leads to photoaddition of psoralen with cutaneous DNA and RNA. Psoralen-UV-A cellular damage may result from the formation of C_4-cycloaddition products of psoralen to DNA and actual intercalation between two base pairs of DNA with formation of strand cross-linkages. (4–6). Psoralens and subsequent exposure to UV-A can lead to inactivation of DNA viruses (7), killing of bacteria (8), and loss of oncogenic potential of neoplastic cells (9). Psoralens and UV-A lead to early inhibition of scheduled DNA synthesis. This has been demonstrated in mouse epidermis (10) and human fibroblast (11) using 8-methoxypsoralen and in male hairless mouse organ culture using trimethylpsoralen (12).

Psoriasis is characterized by a rapidly proliferating epidermis in which the germinative cycle of individual cells is shortened (13). Inhibition of DNA synthesis may be the mechanism by which the psoralen and UV-A combination therapy causes clearing of psoriatic plaques. Topical psoralens and subsequent exposures to UV-A has led to involution of individual psoriatic plaques (3,12,14–16). Multiple treatments are required. Medication must be carefully applied to each individual plaque because in the dose of drug and light used, photosensitization of the normal skin may lead to redness or blistering. As the scaling and induration disappear, marked hyperpigmentation occurs at the site of previously existing psoriatic plaque.

PUVA PHOTOCHEMOTHERAPY OF PSORIASIS

Several hundred patients have now been treated with oral 8-methoxypsoralen and subsequent exposure to UV-A (17–19). Figures 3 and 4 are examples of patients treated with oral psoralen photochemotherapy. Complete clearing occurs in 90% of patients in 8–19 treatments, while another 8% are slow responders (improve considerably but do not completely clear or require 20 or more treatments). Two percent do not respond satisfactorily. A multicenter university trial is being conducted to treat and follow 1600 patients and early reports suggest similar results, although clearing may take somewhat longer because of a conservative protocol of permitted increases in the UV-A doses.

Severe itching (5%), marked redness in localized areas (20%), and

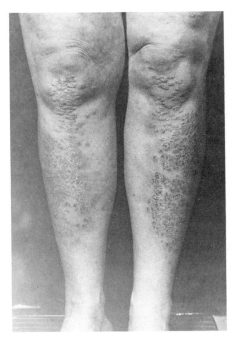 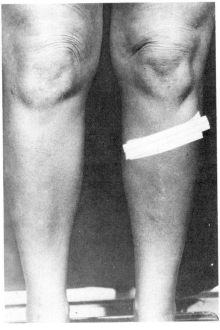

3 Patient with psoriasis vulgaris before and after oral psoralen photochemotherapy.

desquamation (3%) were seen often during the early experience with oral psoralen photochemotherapy but have become less severe and less frequent as more experience is gained and dosimetry becomes more exact. In treatment of the last 100 patients therapy has not been interrupted because of itching or redness (19).

No abnormalities in alkaline phosphatase, serum glutamic oxaloacetic transaminase, complete blood count, urinalysis, bilirubin, or blood urea nitrogen which could be attributed to photochemotherapy were noted in any patient.

PUVA combines the ease of administration of oral medication with the safety of topical medication because the effects are limited to the skin irradiated by UV-A. However, scalp and body folds do not respond if light does not reach those areas. Patients do not have to be hospitalized

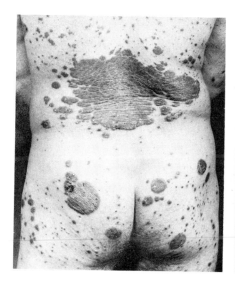
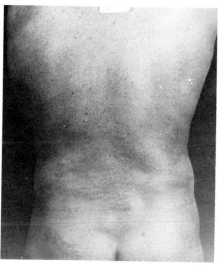

4   Patient with psoriasis vulgaris before and after oral psoralen photochemotherapy.

for therapy. Infrequent treatments are required (two to three times per week) and it appears that weekly maintenance keeps most patients free of psoriasis for months.

The acute limiting factor is erythema which can be avoided by careful dosimetry. In addition, there are several long-term concerns based on animal studies. Long exposure to high-intensity UV-A causes skin cancer and cataracts in laboratory animals. These effects are accelerated by psoralens, especially methoxsalen. Although such effects have not been seen in man in over 20 years of use of methoxsalen and solar UV-A for treatment of vitiligo, careful observation must be maintained. It may be that repeated phototoxic reactions over many years lead to actinic changes in the skin, especially skin which pigments poorly or not at all. The physician must weigh these theoretical risks and the psychological stress of psoriasis against the benefits of effective photochemotherapy. Patients who tan well may actually be proteced by PUVA; the striking psoralen-induced melanogenesis may protect from sunlight and permit less cumulative solar-induced changes over many decades.

LIGHT SOURCE

Besides being electrically safe and having no exposed glass, the ideal light source has the following properties:

(1) *High-intensity UV-A.* Psoralens are activated by UV-A. If large amounts of UV-A energy can be delivered in short periods of time, treatment times are shorter and therefore more practical.

(2) *Omission of "unnecessary" radiation.* The presence of UV-B (sunburn spectrum, 290–320 nm) might lead to erythema-producing reactions before adequate UV-A doses are reached. The presence of excessive infrared radiation causes the skin to become hot and patients feel uncomfortable. These wavebands should be eliminated as much as possible.

(3) *Large field size.* Light sources should be large enough to radiate the entire body surface.

(4) *Uniform intensity with varying distance from the source.* Intensity varies inversely with the square of the distance from a point source of light. For psoralen photochemotherapy such variation would be impractical and dangerous. Light chambers should deliver a known and equal amount to all surfaces of the skin regardless of how close or far from the light. Patients have hips, breasts, noses, chins, and necks; they are not flat sheets of skin and are far from uniform in size.

(5) *Capability of measuring and delivering accurate energy doses.*

DOSIMETRY

Most adults receive 40 mg of 8-MOP (0.6 mg/kg) by mouth 2 hours prior to light exposure. The 2 hour wait is important because cutaneous photosensitivity to UV-A is maximum at 2 hours after ingestion. However, patients do remain photosensitive up to 8 hours after ingestion of the drug.

The dose of light is measured in joules. A joule is an amount of energy (10^7 ergs, work expended by a current of one ampere flowing for 1 second against a resistance of 1 ohm). When speaking of energy one should also specify the unit of area and specify which wavelengths (frequency or photon energy) are being used. A dose frequently used to begin therapy in a tan Caucasian is 3.5 joules/cm² of UV-A (320–400 nm).

Intensity of lamp sources is measured in watts. A watt is simply equal to one joule per second and describes a rate of delivery of energy. A treatment system delivering 10mW/cm² of UV-A would deliver 10 mJ/cm² each second. It would take 350 seconds or 5.83 minutes to deliver 3.5 J/cm² of UV-A with such a treatment system.

SUMMARY

Oral psoralen photochemotherapy is an effective use of a drug plus light combination to treat psoriasis. As long as careful light dosimetry is used it appears to be safe. The long-term side effects are not known but no evidence of serious problems to eye or skin have been noted during decades of experience with the same drug plus sunlight in therapy of skin diseases. The effects of photochemotherapy are limited to the skin because the UV-A required to "activate" the drug does not enter internal organs in appreciable amounts.

REFERENCES

1. M.A. Pathak, D.M. Krämer, and T.B. Fitzpatrick, Photobiology and photochemistry of furocoumarins (psoralens), in "Sunlight and Man: Normal and Abnormal Photobiologic Responses" (M.A. Pathak, L.C. Harber, M. Seiji, and A. Kukita, eds.; T.B. Fitzpatrick, consulting ed.) pp. 335-368. University of Tokyo Press, Tokyo, 1974.
2. M.A. Pathak, F. Daniels, and T.B. Fitzpatrick, The presently known distribution of furocoumarins (psoralens) in plants. *J. Invest. Dermatol.* 39, 225 (1962).
3. K. Toda, M.A. Pathak, J.A. Parrish, and T.B. Fitzpatrick, Alteration of racial differences in melanosome distribution in human epidermis after exposure to ultraviolet. *Nature (New Biol.)* 236, 143 (1972).
4. R.S. Cole, Light-induced cross-linking of DNA in the presence of a furocoumarin (psoralen). *Biochim. Biophys. Acta* 217, 30 (1970).
5. R.S. Cole, Inactivation of *Escherichia coli*, F' Episomes at Transfer and Bacteriophage Lambda by Psoralen plus 360-nm light: Significance of Deoxyribonucleic Acid Cross-Links. *J. Bacteriol.* 107, 846 (1971).
6. F. Dall'Acqua, S. Marciani, L. Ciavatta, and G. Rodighiero, Formation of interstrand cross-linkings in the photoreactions between furocoumarins and DNA. *Z. Naturforsch. (B)* 26, 561 (1971).
7. L. Musajo et al., Photosensitizing furocoumarins: Interaction with DNA and photo-inactivation of DNA containing viruses. *Experientia* 21, 22-24, (1965).

8. E.L. Oginsky et al., Lethal photosensitization of bacteria with 8-methoxypsoralen to longwavelength ultraviolet radiation. *J. Bacteriol.* 78, 821–833 (1959).

9. L. Musajo et al., Photoinactivation of Ehrlich ascites tumor cells *in vitro* obtained with skin photosensitizing furocoumarins. *Experientia* 23, 335–336 (1967).

10. J.H. Epstein and K. Fukuyama, A study of 8-methoxypsoralen (8-MOP) induced phototoxic effects on mammalian epidermal macromolecular synthesis in vivo. *J. Invest. Dermatol.* 54, 350–351 (1970).

11. H.P. Baden, J.A. Parrington, J.D.A. Delhanty et al., DNA synthesis in normal and xeroderma pigmentosum fibroblasts following treatment with 8-methoxypsoralen and longwave ultraviolet light. *Biochim. Biophys. Acta* 262, 247–255 (1972).

12. J.F. Walter, J.J. Voorhees, W.H. Kelsey, and E.A. Duell, Psoralen plus black light inhibits epidermal DNA synthesis. *Arch. Dermatol.* 107, 861–865 (1973).

13. G.D. Weinstein and P. Frost, Abnormal cell proliferation in psoriasis. *J. Invest. Dermatol.* 50, 254–259 (1968).

14. B. Allyn, Studies on phototoxicity in man and laboratory animals. Read before the 21st annual meeting of the American Academy of Dermatology, Chicago, December 1–6, 1962.

15. H. Tronnier and D. Schüle, First results of therapy with long wave UV after photosensitization of skin, *in* (G.O. Schneck, ed.), "Book of Abstracts, Symposia and Contributed Papers, Sixth International Congress on Photobiology," p. 340. Bochum, Germany, 1972.

16. L. Musajo and G. Rodighiero, Studies on the photo-C-cycloaddition reactions between skin photosensitizing furocoumarins and nucleic acids. *Photochem. Photobiol.* 11, 27–35 (1970).

17. J.A. Parrish, T.B. Fitzpatrick, L. Tanenbaum, and M.A. Pathak, Photochemotherapy of psoriasis with oral methoxsalen and longwave ultraviolet light. *N. Eng. J. Med.* 291, 1207–1212 (1974).

18. K. Wolff, T.B. Fitzpatrick, J.A. Parrish et al., Photochemotherapy for psoriasis with orally administered methoxsalen. *Arch. Dermatol.* 112, 943–950 (1976).

19. J.A. Parrish, T.B. Fitzpatrick, K. Wolff, and B.A. Gilchrist, unpublished data.

Recent Advances in Dermatopharmacology

18

A New Tar Gel–Dermatopharmacology and Clinical Efficacy

PETER HEBBORN
DAVID CRAM

PHARMACOLOGY

Vehicle Design

One central fact emerging from recent research in dermatology and pharmacology is that the choice of vehicle for any active agent is crucial to its efficacy. The proper vehicle can enhance a drug's effect and, conversely, the incorrect vehicle can impede its action (1). The dispersion of griseofulvin in PEG 6000, for instance, radically increases absorption after oral administration, with the result that the drug's bioavailability is doubled, allowing the standard dose to be reduced by half (2). In the area of topical steroids, advances in vehicle design and the technology of solubilizing the steroid in the vehicle have improved the bioavailability of some nonfluorinated molecules to the point where they show vasoconstrictor activity rivaling the fluorinated compounds (3,4). One of the key elements, then, to a drug's therapeutic efficacy appears to be its delivery system. In turn, the cornerstone of an optimum delivery system is solubility—as a drug's solubility in the vehicle is enhanced,

197

bioavailability and therapeutic benefit increase to a maximum when optimum solubility is attained. These principles of solubility and vehicle design have been applied to an insoluble material widely used in dermatology—crude coal tar—in order to improve its bioavailability and efficacy. The result has been the incorporation of what appear to be the therapeutic components of tar in a vehicle that is both esthetic and which enables the equivalent of 0.6% crude coal tar to produce the same clinical response usually seen with 5% crude coal tar (CCT) in hydrophilic ointment.

Rationale for Psoriasis Therapy

Psoriasis is a primary condition for which tar therapy is employed, often in conjunction with ultraviolet light. The epidermal thickening and build-up of scales characteristic of this condition, combined with the inherent insolubility of tar, create a formidable obstacle to tar's penetration into the epidermis, where its primary action is believed to occur. Although the precise mechanism of action of tar in the treatment of psoriasis is still not fully defined, one of the commonly recognized benefits of this compound is its photosensitizing effect when combined with UVL (5). Even this theory is controversial, however, since the action spectrum of 5% crude coal tar ranges from 350 to 400 nm, and the usual photosensitivity peak is around 296 nm (6). Some investigators have proposed that tar also has an indirect inhibitory effect on mitotic activity and protein synthesis that would serve to normalize epidermal turnover time in psoriatic lesions (7).

Only 55% of tar's 10,000 or more different constituents have been identified and assigned a probable function in the compound's overall therapeutic role (5). From the empirical use of tar, however, it is recognized that two properties are related proportionately to a tar preparation's clinical efficacy: its phototoxicity and its fluorescence. The greater the photodynamic effect a compound produces, the less exposure to UV light is required to evoke a therapeutic response. Also, fluorescence is a necessary, but not a sufficient, requirement for therapeutic response. The degree of fluorescence the skin exhibits at intervals of time after application of a tar product is an index of its substantivity and depth of penetration.

Experimental Formulations

With these parameters in mind, an attempt was begun to design an esthetic and highly bioavailable tar preparation for the treatment of psoriasis. Clinical efficacy of the order of that seen with 5% crude coal tar was the primary goal, and the preclinical investigational markers employed were phototoxicity and fluorescence. If tar's bioavailability could be enhanced, its efficacy also should be enhanced; dosage strengths might be reduced, providing a concomitant reduction in adverse side effects such as irritation and folliculitis. Furthermore, if the staining and objectional odor and consistency of crude coal tar could be reduced or eliminated, acceptance of the medication by both patients and nursing staff should improve.

Phototoxic Response

The first formulation to be explored was a combination of tar and a keratolytic gel, following Baden's evaluation of a salicylic acid/propylene glycol gel. Baden showed that the benefits of both corticosteroid treatment and tar/UVL therapy were heightened and accelerated when psoriatic scales were removed beforehand with this gel (8). This relatively simple combination of 3% tar with 6% salicyclic acid and 60% propylene glycol proved to be too phototoxic. Consequently, several reformulations were examined for toxicity and then assessed for photodynamism and fluorescence, first in guinea pigs and later in human volunteers.

In a preliminary screening, using a limited number of albino guinea pigs, it was found that a formulation of propylene glycol (30%), ethyl alcohol (30%), water (26%), and an extract of coal tar (2%; equivalent to 0.6% crude coal tar) elicited nearly as great a phototoxic response as 5% CCT in hydrophilic petrolatum or 1% 8-methoxypsoralen, both well-known topical photosensitizers (Fig. 1) (9). The materials were applied in measured amounts to four shaved and depilated test sites. One site received the test formula, one site 8-methoxypsoralen, and two sites 5% CCT in hydrophilic petrolatum. The compounds were allowed to remain on the skin for 30 minutes and then were removed with olive oil. One CCT site was shielded with cardboard which was taped to the skin, and the other three sites were exposed through window glass to a bank of four Westinghouse FS40 BL type lights for 1 hour at a distance of 10 cm. Visual assessment of the resulting erythema and edema was made 24 hours after exposure and ranked on a scale of 0 to 4, with 4 representing the most severe erythema. The average readings were 2.5 for CCT sites, 2.2 for 8-methoxypsoralen sites, and 1.9 for the tar gel sites. Since the tar gel was found to possess significant phototoxicity when compared to 8-methoxypsoralen and crude coal tar, it was decided to evaluate it in relation to the leading marketed products in a similar

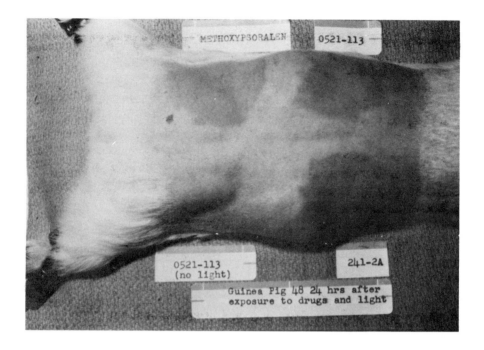

1   Guinea pig photosensitization assay. 241-2A: Tar gel. 0521-113: 5% CCT in hydrophilic ointment.

assay. None of the tested preparations proved to be as photodynamic as the investigational drug (Table I).

In a similar experimental design with human volunteers, this tar gel formula produced a photosensitizing effect equivalent to 5% crude coal tar in hydrophilic ointment (Table II). In addition to ranking high in the photosensitizing assay, this formula was also considered more pleasant to use than crude coal tar by the subjects. (It subsequently was given the name "Estar[TM],"[a] to convey the fact of its esthetic qualities in contrast to crude coal tar.)

In the meantime, various other tar preparations were evaluated by Tanenbaum and his associates in a more sophisticated system (10). They

---

[a] Estar[TM] gel supplied by Westwood Pharmaceuticals, Inc.

Table I. Guinea Pig Photodynamism Assay

Product	Mean erythema reading[a]
Tar gel	2.75
Zetar	2.19
Iocon	1.75
Tar Doak lotion	1.57
Ionil T	0.63
Pentrax	0.05

[a]0-4 scale.

Table II. Photodynamism on Human Arms, following UVA Irradiation

Compound	Mean erythema reading[a]
5% cct in H.O.	3.00 (standard)
Tar gel	3.00
Zetar	2.00
Tar Doak lotion	0.38
Alphosyl gel	0.00
Alphosyl lotion	0.13
Iocon	0.00
Ionil T	0.00
Pentrax	0.00

[a]0-4 scale.

measured the minimum dose of UVA (joules/sq cm) required to produce a phototoxic response in humans treated with standard amounts of selected preparations 1 hour prior to exposure. They reported that the mean phototoxic dose for 5% CCT in petrolatum was 7.8 ± 3.0 joules/sq cm. In this bioassay system, tar gel required 4.0 joules/sq cm for a phototoxic response (11). This comparison showed that less UVA energy is required to produce a therapeutic phototoxic response 1 hour after treatment with the tar gel than is required with the other tested tar preparations, including 5% crude coal tar. Kaidbey and Kligman had earlier reported that the intensity of phototoxic response from coal tar preparations is strongly influenced by the base (12). These data suggested that the use of this gel base was contributing significantly to

Table III. Substantivity: Fluorescence on Human Skin[a]

Product	Days following application				
	0[b]	1	2	3	4
Tar gel	3.75	2.50	1.85	0.65	0.35
Zetar	2.80	1.35	0.40	0.10	0.10
Pentrax	3.0	0.35	0	0	0
Tar Doak lotion	3.25	0.12	0	0	0
Alphosyl gel	1.30	0	0	0	0
Alphosyl lotion	1.30	0	0	0	0

[a]0-4 scale.
[b]0, is the fluorescence noted one hour after application.

the preparation's biological activity—so much so that it was comparable to the standard tar products used in hospital practice, which contain crude coal tar at a higher percentage than the extract used in this formula.

Penetration

One interesting phenomenon noted during these assays was that, with some preparations, the photosensitizing effect seemed to persist for 48 hours or longer after initial application to skin and this could have considerable clinical significance. As a simple means of quantitating the duration of the tar's activity, a series of fluorescence assays was set up. Seven different tar preparations were applied to the forearms of human volunteers, allowed to remain for 5 minutes and then rinsed off. Visual readings of relative fluorescence (rated on a scale of 0 to 4) were made 1 hour after application and daily thereafter for 4 days. After 24 hours, three of the test compounds showed virtually no fluorescence—they had almost completely washed off the surface of the skin (Table III). The tar gel alone continued to produce more than minimal fluorescence at day 4. This indicated that the tar gel was substantive to the skin to a greater degree than the other tar formulations in the assay.

To judge the relative depth of penetration into human skin achieved by the tar gel and 5% CCT, serial stripping of the stratum corneum was employed, in conjunction with fluorescence readings. Measured amounts of the test materials were applied to the backs of volunteers; 1 hour after application, successive layers of stratum corneum cells were removed with cellophane tape. Fluorescent material present in stripped cell layers was extracted in alcohol and measured with a Turner Fluorometer. The first layer of stratum corneum from the 5% CCT in hydrophilic ointment-treated sites exhibited eight times more fluorescence than did skin treated with the tar gel. This corresponds to the relative degrees of fluorescence of the two preparations *in vitro*. As successive layers were stripped and analyzed for fluorescence, the CCT preparation continued to show greater activity than the tar gel. At about the twentieth layer the two formulas began to become equivalent (Fig. 2). Other products tested showed no fluorescence after 4 or 5 strips, which indicates they essentially remained at the surface of the stratum corneum. Although this assay only reflects penetration of the stratum corneum, it can be taken as an indication of potential therapeutic efficacy, since the former is a prerequisite for penetration into the epidermis.

The clinical efficacy of the tar gel has been evaluated over the past 2 years in a variety of therapeutic regimens ranging from the complex Goeckerman method to simple daily application with no other form of treatment. The following section describes the results of one segment of this clinical evaluation.

CLINICAL EXPERIENCE (13)

From March 1974 to March 1975, 60 patients with psoriasis were treated at the University of California, San Francisco, with the new tar gel and ultraviolet light in a modified Goeckerman regimen (13). As experience with the agent increased, paired comparisons with crude coal tar were made. The cosmetic qualities of the tar gel made it suitable also for use in outpatients with psoriasis and atopic eczema; in some cases topical corticosteroids and keratolytic agent also were used.

Methods and Materials

Sixty patients with extensive psoriasis who either were hospitalized or were being treated in the San Francisco Day Care Center for Psoriasis received applications of the tar gel three times a day, followed by increasing erythemal doses of ultraviolet light once a day. The tar gel was applied to all body surfaces, including intertriginous areas, and also to the scalp in some patients. In 10 patients the tar gel was applied to half the body and 2% crude coal tar in petrolatum to the other half in order to provide a paired comparison. The medications were applied by hand by a nurse. The patients were bathed once a day, with liberal

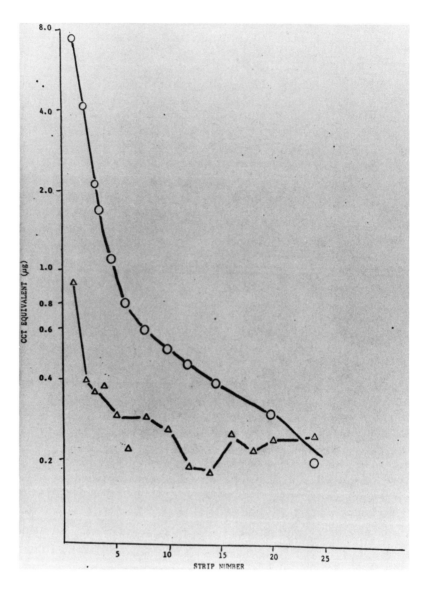

2

Penetration of tar products into human epidermis (stripped 1 hour after application). O—O. 5% CTT in hydrophilic ointment; △—△, tar gel.

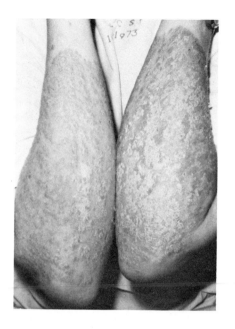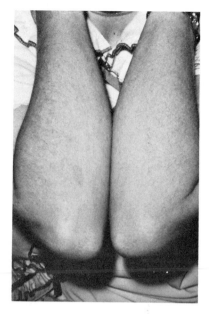

3

Clearing of psoriasis of the forearms after 3 weeks of tar gel and ultraviolet light. (Cram, DL: Treatment of psoriasis with tar gel. *Cutis* 17, 1197-1203 (1976).

amounts of bath oil added to the water, and a bland lubricant was applied at night to keep the skin moist.

The ultraviolet light source was 12 commercially available fluorescent sunlamp bulbs which produce a continuous output spectrum between 275 and 380 nm, with a broad peak at 313 nm (UVB). The bulbs were mounted in an upright cabinet in which the patients stood during their treatment.

To investigate the possibility of a synergistic effect with multiple medications, we applied a steroid ointment (fluocinonide 0.5%) and a potent keratolytic (6% salicylic acid in 60% propylene glycol), in addition to the tar gel, to heavy plaques in several patients. A number of outpatients with psoriasis and a few with atopic eczema were treated with the tar gel both alone and in combination with hydrocortisone cream (1%).

Results and Discussion

Of 60 inpatients with psoriasis, 50 experienced good to excellent results: complete or nearly complete clearing was accomplished in 2 to 4 weeks (Figs. 3, 4). The patients in whom fair results or no changes

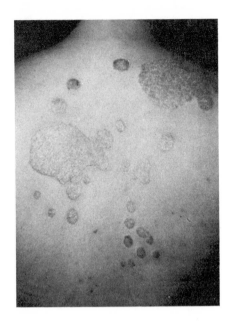

4   Clearing of psoriasis of the back after 3 weeks of tar gel and ultraviolet light. (Cram, DL: Treatment of psoriasis with a tar gel. *Cutis* 17, 1197-1203 (1976).

were reported were those for whom the tar gel was too drying or produced irritation, which they described as burning or stinging. For the most part, these were elderly patients. No allergic contact sensitivity was observed in any of the patients treated. Table IV summarizes the results from the inpatient group.

In the paired comparison studies, the 2% crude coal tar in petrolatum produced a somewhat quicker therapeutic response than did the tar gel in nearly all patients treated. In addition, the side treated with the tar gel developed more erythema than the crude coal tar side; this difference may have been due to either the greater photodynamic effect of the tar gel or the protective petrolatum vehicle of the crude coal tar. We have not observed a significant difference in the dose of ultraviolet light necessary to produce a therapeutic response in patients treated with the tar gel versus those treated with crude coal tar. However, some patients have reported a greater sensitivity to natural sunlight while using the tar gel. They developed significant discomfort and ultraviolet reactions

Table IV. Sixty Psoriasis Inpatients

Response[a]	Number of patients
Excellent	40
Good	10
Fair	7
No change	3
Worse	0

[a]Clearing time: 2-4 weeks

in treated areas that were exposed to intense natural sunlight, even after cleansing those sites. This effect may be due to the tar gel's greater substantivity or to its photodynamic qualities. Patients should be cautioned about exposure to strong sunlight while using this medication.

The tar gel also was observed to produce a unique exfoliative effect as it cleared the psoriatic plaques. This progressive peeling of the plaques at first appeared to be a worsening of the condition, until it was recognized as a part of the clearing process. This exfoliative effect appears as early as a few days after the tar gel applications are begun, and gradually lessens as the plaques flatten. Lubricating ointments help prevent this scaling and do not seem to reduce the effectiveness of the tar gel.

All patients who tolerated the medication preferred the tar gel to crude coal tar, largely because of its cosmetic qualities—ease of application, mild tar odor, and negligible staining potential. Stains can be avoided by rubbing the gel well into the skin, allowing a few minutes for it to dry, and removing any excess by patting with a tissue. Any stains that inadvertently do occur can be washed out easily. Folliculitis, an occasional complication of tar therapy, was rarely observed with the tar gel. Nearly all outpatients with psoriasis who were treated with the tar gel showed excellent responses, even without the use of ultraviolet light, and acceptance of the medication by patients was uniformly excellent.

It is recognized that the Goeckerman regimen and its variants can produce long remissions (14,15). Our experience with the tar gel in this regimen is too brief, however, to compare the length of remission following this latest modification with that which follows crude coal tar applications and ultraviolet light.

The effect of the tar gel appeared to be enhanced by the addition of

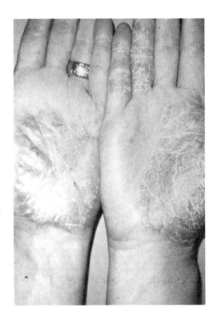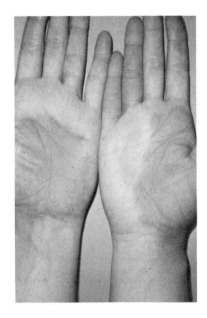

5
Psoriasis of palms and fingers with significant clearing after 2 weeks of tar gel, keratolytic gel, and topical corticosteroid. (Cram, DL: Treatment of psoriasis with a tar gel. *Cutis*, 17, 1197-1203 (1976).

fluocinonide ointment and, in some patients with thick plaques, a keratolytic gel. The skin was first hydrated by bathing, and then the keratolytic gel was applied; this was followed by the tar gel and the corticosteroid, each three times a day. With this combination, plaques often cleared completely in 2 to 3 weeks; this regimen was found especially useful on psoriasis of the palms and soles (Fig. 5). Also significant was the nearly uniform effectiveness of the tar gel plus hydrocortisone cream in intertriginous areas, without the production of folliculitis. Scalp psoriasis, however, responded less well to the tar gel.

The few atopic eczema patients who were treated with this medication and lubricants showed improvement. The gel was discontinued in a few patients because of its drying effect. More experience is needed in our evaluation of this medication in eczema patients.

Table V. Advantages and Disadvantages of Tar Gel

Advantages	Disadvantages
Superior cosmetic qualities	Response slower than crude coal
negligible staining	tar in some patients
mild tar odor	Can be drying without lubrication
easy to apply	Produced irritation in some
Rarely produced folliculitis	patients
Approaches crude coal tar in	
efficacy	
Effective without UVL	
Effectiveness enhanced by keratolytics	
and corticosteroids	
Excellent outpatient treatment	

SUMMARY

Our year of clinical experience with this new tar gel has shown it to be effective for psoriasis in a variety of therapeutic regimens. Good to excellent results were obtained when it was used (1) with ultraviolet light in a modified Goeckerman regimen, (2) without ultraviolet light, (3) with prior application of a keratolytic agent, and (4) with concomitant applications of steroids.

Along with its therapeutic effectiveness, this new tar gel also largely overcomes the objectionable features of previous tar preparations: it is easy to apply, has only a mild tar odor, and has negligible staining potential. The advantages and disadvantages of the tar gel are summarized in Table V. As can be seen, this unique medication not only appears to deliver all of the customary benefits of crude coal tar, but it does so in a form that is convenient to apply and cosmetically acceptable.

REFERENCES

1. J.W. Hadgraft, Recent progress in the formulation of vehicles for topical applications. *Br. J. Dermatol.* 87, 386–390 (1972).
2. W.L. Chiou and S. Riegelman, Absorption characteristics of solid dispersed and micronized griseofulvin in man. *J. Pharm. Sci.* 60, 1376–1380 (1971).

3. J. Almeyda and B.W. Burt, Double blind controlled study of treatment of atopic eczema with a preparation of hydrocortisone in a new drug delivery system versus betamethasone 17-valerate. *Br. J. Dermatol.* 91, 579–583 (1974).

4. M. Whitefield and A.W. McKenzie, A new formulation of 0.1% hydrocortisone cream with vasoconstrictor activity and clinical effectiveness. *Br. J. Dermatol.* 92, 585–588 (1975).

5. C. Grupper, The chemistry, pharmacology, and use of tar in the treatment of psoriasis. *Psoriasis, Proc. Int. Symp.*, E.M. Farber and A.J. Cox (eds.), pp. 347–356. Stanford P. Press 1971.

6. M.A. Everett and J.V. Miller, Coal tar and ultraviolet light: II Cumulative effects. *Arch. Dermatol.* 84, 937–940 (1961).

7. J. Ruzicka, V. Novotna-Kasparkova, and V. Burda, Die wirkung von teerpaste und yperisalbe auf den oxydativen glucosestoffwechsel in der psoriatischen haut. *Arch. Klin. Exp. Derm.* 234, 175–181 (1969).

8. H.P. Baden, Treatment of hyperkeratotic dermatitis of the palms. *Arch. Dermatol.* 110, 737–738 (1974).

9. L.C. Harber, personal communication.

10. L. Tanenbaum, J.A. Parrish, M.A. Pathak, R.R. Anderson, and T.B. Fitzpatrick, Tar phototoxicity and phototherapy for psoriasis. *Arch. Dermatol.* 111, 467–470 (1975).

11. H.P. Baden, personal communication.

12. K.H. Kaidbey and A.M. Kligman, Topical photosensitizers. *Arch. Dermatol.* 110, 868–870 (1974).

13. D.L. Cram, Treatment of psoriasis with a tar gel. *Cutis*, 17, 1197–1203 (1976).

14. H.O. Perry, C.W. Soderstron, and R.W. Schulze, The Goeckerman treatment of psoriasis. *Arch. Dermatol.* 98, 178–182 (1968).

15. D.L. Cram, Psoriasis day care center. *Int. J. Dermatol.* 14, 577–578 (1975).

19

Modulation of Keratinization with α-Hydroxy Acids and Related Compounds

EUGENE J. VAN SCOTT
RUEY J. YU

The possibility of therapeutic control of what have been called disorders of keratinization has been tied to finding agents that either restrain excessive keratinization or agents that "normalize" what might be considered faulty keratinization. A rather long list of cutaneous disorders would seem to be possibly benefited by such agents: e.g., psoriasis, where keratinization is incomplete in association with rapid transit of cells through the epidermis; acne, where keratinization of follicular orifices is such that keratinized cells are retained to form obstructive comedones; the ichthyosiform dermatoses, where the stratum corneum is abnormally keratinized resulting in fine scaling such as in ichthyosis vulgaris, or is "hyperkeratinized" and its exfoliation delayed such as in lamellar ichthyosis; and an array of dermatoses where stratum corneum formation departs from normal to one degree or another and accounts for a major clinical expression of the disease.

A paramount need in the search for such agents has been a reliable screening system to identify those having a specific influence on keratinization. In earlier studies we have explored the suitability of the skin of the rhino mouse, a variant of the hairless mouse with extraordinary epidermal hyperkeratinization, to evaluate the "antikeratinization" activity of topically applied candidate materials (1). Vitamin A acid, topically applied to the skin of this animal consistently restores keratinization to normal appearing states, but other materials usually considered to have an influence on keratinization, e.g., salicylic acid, fail to have a demonstratable normalizing effect. Thus, after testing hundreds of chemical agents on this animal we have judged the screening system to be inadequate due to its apparent limitation of specificity for vitamin A materials alone.

Several patients with ichthyosiform dermatoses, seeking relief from their affliction that had not been obtainable by the few inadequate conventional remedies available, provided the circumstance for a search of improved treatments of their particular dermatosis. This search fortuitously led to the finding that a group of α-hydroxy acids and related chemicals when topically applied in 5–10% concentrations in cream or ointment vehicles rather consistently abrogated the features of hyperkeratinization in most of these dermatoses, restoring toward normal the clinical and histologic appearance of the skin so treated (2). This group of compounds included citric acid, glycolic acid, glucuronic acid, 3-hydroxybutyric acid, 2-hydroxyisobutyric acid, lactic acid, malic acid, pyruvic acid, ethyl and methyl pyruvates, tartaric acid, and tartronic acid.

The efficacy of these compounds on these dermatoses have been repeatedly confirmed by us and, since our initial report, we have found additional compounds having structural and metabolic similarities to possess similar functional influences on keratinization in ichthyosis vulgaris and lamellar ichthyosis when also applied in 5–10% concentrations. This group of compounds include α-hydroxybutyric acid, cysteic acid, homocysteic acid, galacturonic acid, gluconolactone, glucuronolactone, mucic acid, β-phenyllactic acid, β-phenylpyruvic acid, and saccharic acid.

Although in our initial observations (2) we concluded that the type of vehicle was not a major determinant of final effectiveness of preparations, our further experience leads us to prefer oil-in-water vehicles, such as hydrophilic ointment USP insofar as desquamation of the thickened stratum corneum occurs more rapidly than with water-in-oil vehicles. The reason for this is not entirely clear however.

All the foregoing compounds are comparable in their efficacy on the ichthyotic disorders with seeming minor differences from case to case. Because of an initial large supply of glycolic acid, we have preferentially utilized formulations containing this chemical. Figures 1 and

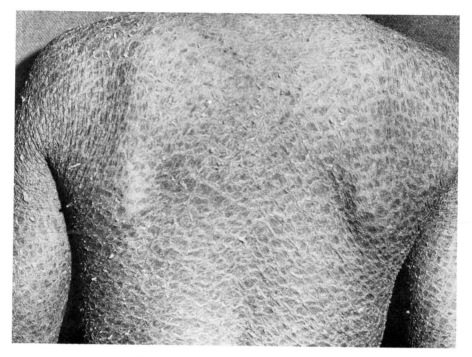

1 Back of 10-year-old boy with lamellar ichthyosis prior to treatment.

2 illustrate the kind of response usually obtainable in lamellar ichthyosis. The effects on keratinization of these materials do not appear limited to the ichthyotic disorders, although the parameters for measuring effects in other disorders of keratinization are not so precise as in the ichthyoses. Effects on follicular hyperkeratinization were suggested by changes observed in the skin of patients with lamellar ichthyosis, where follicular plugging is quite characteristic (3). Figures 3 and 4 illustrate that in such cases hyperkeratinization within follicular orifices is restrained by the α-hydroxy acids in a manner similar to that on the epidermal surface, although the effects on the follicles may not be so promptly manifested. The potential efficacy of these materials on the topical management of acne vulgaris, and whether beneficial effects can be sustained over long periods, requires more detailed study. Our early

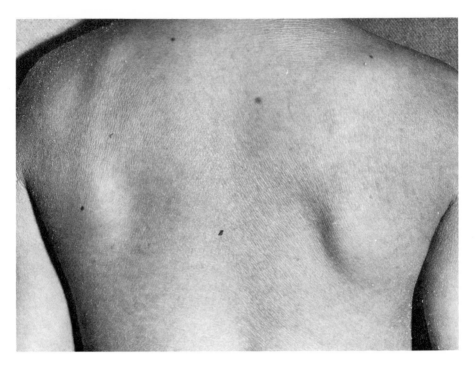

2 After 2 weeks of b.i.d. topical application of 5% glycolic acid in hydrophilic ointment USP skin is clinically normal in appearance.

observations nevertheless indicate that these compounds influence keratinization in a number of skin disorders.

Analyses of blood and urine from one of our patients with lamellar ichthyosis showed that while the pyruvic acid content was normal in the blood (0.103 mM) and low in the urine (0.133 mM), the lactic acid content was normal in the blood (0.985 mM) and very low in the urine (0.079mM). The lactic acid concentration in the normal human skin is reported to be three times or more that in the blood, due to glycolytic enzymes such as hexokinase, phosphofructokinase, and lactic dehydrogenase which actively convert glucose to lactic acid in the epidermis (4).

A fundamental question concerns the means by which this group of chemicals, most of which are physiologic in humans, exert what might be termed pharmacologic effects on keratinization. The fact that a

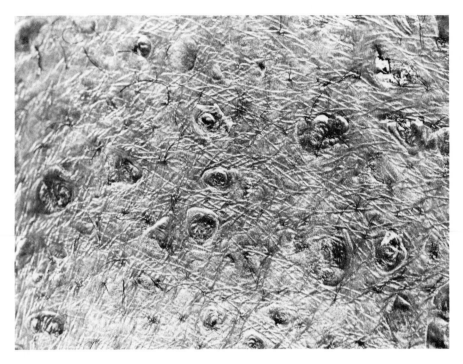

3 Anterior thigh of patient with lamellar ichthyosis after 2 weeks topical treatment with 5% glycolic acid cream. Although surface stratum corneum appears normal, follicular plugging   persists.

patient with lamellar ichthyosis with a normal range of lactate content in his blood responds beneficially to the topical administration of lactic acid suggests that the epidermis in his skin is either producing insufficient amounts or eliminating too much lactate from the epidermis. It is, however, still not known whether or not the higher concentration of lactate in the skin has any important role in the feedback control of the glycolytic pathway or other metabolic pathways in normal keratinization of the epidermis.

Refsum's syndrome is also a hereditary disorder but is characterized by neurologic abnormalities and may be accompanied by exceptional dryness and scaling of skin clinically similar to ichthyosis. It has been shown that patients having Refsum's disease accumulate large stores (fifty-fold or greater) of phytanic acid in their blood and tissues, such as viscera and brain (5). Studies on fibroblasts from patients suffering

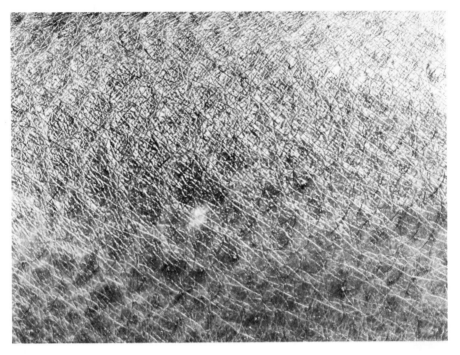

4   Same site as in Fig. 3, after an additional 2 weeks of topical therapy with 5% glycolic acid. Follicular hyperkeratinization is no longer discernible.

from Refsum's disease suggest that the excessive accumulation of phytanic acid is due to a defect in a single enzyme system which converts phytanic acid to α-hydroxyphytanic acid (6). It is, however, still not known what role α-hydroxyphytanic acid plays in skin with regard to normal keratinization.

Although more basal cells in the epidermis of patients with lamellar ichthyosis and epidermolytic hyperkeratosis are in mitosis, this is not the case in ichthyosis vulgaris and X-linked ichthyosis. The common major defect in the ichthyoses therefore might be due to a delay in the exfoliation of the stratum corneum. Mucopolysaccharides are reported to serve as the intercellular cementing substance for normal keratinization of the epidermis (7). It remains to be seen whether physiologic

α-hydroxy acids such as lactic acid and α-hydroxyphytanic acid might play key roles in the biosynthesis of mucopolysaccharides.

SUMMARY

Alphahydroxy acids and certain related chemicals, most of which are physiologic in human tissues, when topically applied to the skin of patients with ichthyotic disorders restore keratinization to clinically normal states. The mechanism of action of these chemicals on keratinization is not yet clarified. One or more metabolic pathways may be involved, perhaps those involved are the biosyntheses of mucopolysaccharides.

REFERENCES

1. E.J. Van Scott, Experimental animal integumental models for screening potential dermatologic drugs, in "Pharmacology and the Skin," (W. Montagna, E.J. Van Scott, and R.B. Stoughton, eds.), pp. 523–533. New York, Meredith Corporation, 1972.
2. E.J. Van Scott and R.J. Yu, Control of keratinization with α-hydroxy acids and related compounds. I. Topical treatment of ichthyotic disorders. *Arch. Derm.* 110, 586–590 (1974).
3. P. Frost and E.J. Van Scott, Ichthyosiform dermatoses. *Arch. Derm.* 94, 113–126 (1966).
4. J.A. Johnson and R.M. Fusaro, The role of the skin in carbohydrate metabolism in "Advances in Metabolic Disorders." R. Levine and R. Luft (eds.), Vol. 6, pp. 1–55. New York, Academic Press Inc., 1972.
5. D. Steinberg, J.H. Herndon, Jr., B.W. Uhlendorf, C.E. Mize, J. Avigan, and G.W.A. Milne, Refsum's Disease: Nature of the enzyme defect. *Science* 156, 1740–1742 (1967).
6. J.H. Herndon, Jr., D. Steinberg, B.W. Uhlendorf, and H.M. Fales, Refsum's disease: Characterization of the enzyme defect in cell culture. *J. Clin. Invest.* 48, 1017–1032 (1969).
7. E.H. Mercer, R.A. Jahn, and H.I. Maibach, Surface coats containing polysaccharides on human epidermal cells. *J. Invest. Dermatol.* 51, 204–214 (1968).

Recent Advances in Dermatopharmacology

20

The Management of Hyperkeratosis

HOWARD P. BADEN

The stratum corneum is a complex multilayered structure formed during the final stages of keratinization in the epidermis. The microscopic appearance of the stratum corneum is similar on most areas of the body except for a variation in thickness (1). One observes that the cornified cells are aligned in very orderly stacks and that cells in neighboring stacks show very precise overlapping of their edges (2). This produces a rather tightly organized physical membrane rather well suited to the barrier function of the stratum corneum. The stratum corneum of the palms and soles has a quite different appearance and does not show the same orderly arrangement of cells.

The stratum corneum is highly insoluble and can only be dissolved by aqueous solutions containing denaturing agents. One may view this resistance as an intracellular or intercellular phenomenon. The components within the cell are responsible for maintaining cellular integrity while the intercellular materials work to cement the cells to one another.

A major component of the epidermal cell is the α fibrous protein which appears as filaments in the electronmicrographs of the skin. These filaments are first observed in the basal layer and go through a series of

Table I.

Amino acids	Prekeratin
Lysine	5.1
Histidine	1.0
Arginine	6.1
Aspartic acid	9.1
Threonine	4.0
Serine	11.1
Glutamic acid	14.1
Proline	1.4
Glycine	16.4
Alanine	6.7
Valine	4.0
Methionine	1.3
Isoleucine	3.5
Leucine	9.2
Tyrosine	2.8
Phenylalanine	3.6
Half cystine	0.6

changes as the cells ascend into the stratum corneum. It is thought that these 70–80 Å filaments extend across the cell from one wall to another hooking on to attachment plates of desmosomes. Since it has been estimated that the basic fibrous protein has a length which is only a fraction of the width of a cell, the filaments must result from an aggregation of fibrous proteins. The fibrous protein has been shown to be a helical molecule, similar but not identical to the classical α helix.

The α proteins have been most extensively studied in cow snout epidermis (3–5). The α protein of the viable epidermis, prekeratin, can be solubilized by urea or buffers of organic acids below pH 2.7. Purification from acid buffers can be achieved by isoelectric precipitation. This material is insoluble at the pH range 3–10, but can be maintained in solution at neutral pH by the addition of urea, guanidine, or sodium dodecyl sulfate (SDS). Amino acid analysis reveals a high content of the acidic amino acids and glycine (Table I). The cystine content is quite low, unlike the α protein of hair and nail. Electrophoresis in SDS has shown a number of components (Fig. 1) and immunologic studies indicate that the A and B families are distinct, but both are necessary to form an α helix. These results are best interpreted as the prekeratin molecule consisting of 3 polypeptides, two A and one B chain. It would

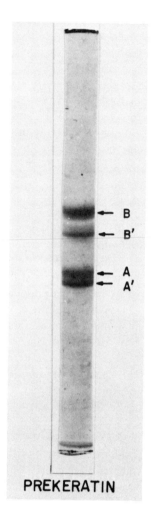

1

SDS polyacrylamide electrophoresis
of prekeratin. The direction
of electrophoresis is down.

PREKERATIN

appear that there is a major prekeratin with the chains A, A′, B, and a
minor one with an A, A′, and B′. No cystine cross-links occur between
the polypeptides of prekeratin.

As the cells of the viable epidermis become cornified at the base of
the stratum corneum the α fibrous proteins become cross-linked and can
only be solubilized by alkaline buffers containing a denaturing agent
such as urea and a reducing agent (6, 7). This process is irreversible
and the stratum corneum fibrous proteins become cross-linked when the

reducing agent is removed. The amino acid composition of the stratum corneum reveals a ½-cystine content of 2 residues/100 residues indicating that no ½ cystine rich matrix proteins are present as has been found in hair and nail (8).

Thus, the system for maintaining the integrity of the epidermal cells in the stratum corneum involves filamentous protein which is attached to the cell wall and which shows interchain-disulfide cross-linkage. Another structural protein complex, keratohyalin, unique to the epidermis also is involved. This material is newly synthesized in the granular layer and has been thought to coat the filaments and stabilize them. The controversy which exists concerning the chemical nature of the material probably has as its basis the complex nature of the material and the different methods used by several investigators to isolate it (9,10). It has been difficult, however, to accept the function of keratohyalin since in a number of conditions including ichthyosis vulgaris no keratohyalin is formed, yet the filaments and stratum corneum appear to be normally stabilized. More work is necessary to determine the exact role of keratohyalin.

A final unique feature of the keratinization process is the deposition of a lipid material between the filaments (11). X-ray diffraction studies have indicated that a polar lipid with its long axis perpendicular to that of the filaments appears as cornification procedes. It is likely that this protein-lipid-complex functions as the barrier. Extraction of the stratum corneum with lipid solvents removes the lipid and at the same time the barrier function of the stratum corneum is lost.

What has been described may be called the intracellular cement materials and probably is the major barrier of the stratum corneum. Our preliminary work with human epidermis and that of other animals indicates that what has been found in bovine snout epidermis is generally applicable. As research continues in this area new facts will be added to complete the picture.

Information on intercellular cement is far less complete. In the viable epidermis no irreversible linkage between cells can be present since cells move up from the basal layer to the stratum corneum. The desmosomes of the epidermis are clearly important in holding cells together and when these are disturbed as in certain diseases acantholysis or cell separation and blistering occurs (12). As a cell rises in the epidermis these attachments must constantly be broken and reformed. The mechanism for this process has not been clarified.

A carbohydrate material called glycocalyx (13) has been described coating keratinocytes in the viable epidermis. This material may be the antigen which reacts with the antibody found in the sera of patients with pemphigus. What role this material plays in holding cells together remains to be demonstrated.

In the stratum corneum a firm attachment between cells is formed. This is in part a result of the stacking which has been observed which permits careful overlapping of cells and maximum use of cell surfaces (2). The thickness of the stratum corneum is almost certainly related to the capacity of cells to stick together. Eventually at the skin surface loss of cell adhesion occurs and desquamation results. By inference from what has been observed in certain forms of ichthyosis the ability of cells to hold together is inversely related to the water content of the stratum corneum. Thus, the common type of winter dry skin frequently ameliorates when the individual is exposed to a high humidity environment.

Hyperkeratosis, or thickening of the stratum corneum can result from exposure of normal epidermis to a variety of stimuli including pressure, ultraviolet rays, and chemicals. This may result in significant symptoms for which the patient will seek medical help, such as with calluses of the soles. For the most part, however, thickening of the stratum corneum is a partial or major expression of some disease process. Although one tends to think of the genetic diseases such as ichthyosis as representing the major cause of hyperkeratosis, the common dermatoses such as seborrheic dermatitis, eczema and psoriasis are most commonly at fault.

The management of hyperkeratosis can be directed to modification of the pathogenetic mechanism leading to the accumulation of increased amounts of stratum corneum. Inhibition of increased cellular replication by chemotherapeutic agents such as the use of methotrexate in psoriasis is an example of this (14). With the return of the epidermis to its normal rate of turnover, accumulation of an abnormally thick stratum corneum may cease and the hyperkeratosis will disappear.

In the case of topical therapeutic agents the thickened stratum corneum may limit penetration of the drug which could return the diseased skin to a normal state. At first fortuitously and now more deliberately many vehicles are designed to help in the breakdown of the stratum corneum. This is particularly true when occlusion with plastic dressings is part of the treatment.

This brings us to the second method of managing hyperkeratosis, which is the use of agents that remove thickened stratum corneum. The term keratolysis has been used to describe this phenomenon which for the most part is a softening and peeling of the stratum corneum rather than a true dissolution. Blank (15) recognized that softening of the stratum corneum resulted from hydration of the skin and when prolonged could lead to disintegration of the stratum corneum. This can be observed as an experiment of nature by noting the improvement in such conditions as dominant and sex-linked ichthyosis when the affected individual is placed in a warm humid environment.

The traditional keratolytic agent over the years has been salicylic acid in concentrations up to 6% in a variety of cream and ointment vehicles (16). The more hydrophobic preparations appeared most effective but were messy to use.

The more recent developments in keratolytic therapy resulted from the observation that a steroid preparation containing propylene glycol was exceptionally effective in scale removal. A controlled study was undertaken in patients with ichthyosis vulgaris and sex-linked ichthyosis to ascertain the effectiveness of propylene glycol and water mixtures in removing stratum corneum (17). Excellent results occurred in sex-linked ichthyosis after two to three applications of 60% propylene glycol under occlusion, with removal of the dark adherent scales. The treatment was repeated intermittently as needed. In ichthyosis vulgaris the results were similar with 60% of the patients experiencing complete clearing while the other 40% of the patients had varying degrees of improvement.

Occlusion without the propylene glycol had only minimal effect while the use of propylene glycol without occlusion gave less than optimal improvement. The optimal concentraion of propylene glycol was 60% since this gave maximal keratolysis with minimal irritation. Significant keratolysis, however, could be demonstrated with concentrations as low as 40%. Irritation was a minor complaint in some patients and was rapidly relieved by stopping the treatment for a day.

Attempts to develop a preparation that would be effective without occlusion were not successful. Propylene glycol was incorporated into a variety of hydrophobic and hydrophilic ointments with and without water, and these preparations were applied to the skin of patients with ichthyosis vulgaris and sex-linked ichthyosis two to three times a day. Although the preparations produced temporary smoothness of the skin, significant removal of the thickened stratum corneum could not be appreciated even when the preparations were used for several weeks.

Although the propylene glycol water mixture was an effective form of therapy it was not entirely satisfactory in some patients with ichthyosis vulgaris and lamellar ichthyosis. Since salicylic acid was known to be an effective keratolytic agent, a study was undertaken to determine if it would increase the potency of the propylene glycol solution (18).

Table II. Response of Ichthyosis to the Keratolytic Gel[a]

Disease	Response	Occluded	Not occluded
Ichthyosis vulgaris	None	1	3
	Moderate	2	9
	Marked	5	12
	Clear	21	0
Sex-linked ichthyosis	None	0	1
	Moderate	0	4
	Marked	0	1
	Clear	6	0
Lamellar ichthyosis	None	1	5
	Moderate	2	0
	Marked	2	0
	Clear	0	0

[a]One side was treated with occlusion and the other without. Some of the patients with ichthyosis vulgaris occluded both sides because they felt it was more effective, resulting in fewer patients in the not occluded category.

Because of the limited solubility of the acid, alcohol had to be added as a solvent. The optimal formulation contained 6% salicylic acid, 20% ethanol, and 20% water in propylene glycol.

This preparation was very effective in removing thickened stratum corneum from ichthyosis vulgaris, sex-linked ichthyosis, and lamellar ichthyosis, especially when occlusive dressings were used. Omission of salicylic acid from the preparation demonstrated that the salicylic acid rather than the alcohol was the potentiating agent. The liquid preparation was not so well accepted by patients because it had a tendency to run and produced irritations when it collected in skin folds. The difficulty was overcome by a gel formulation which received excellent patient acceptance. In paired comparison studies the gel was equally as effective as the solution.

The keratolytic gel proved to be an effective agent for removal of scales in ichthyosis vulgaris as shown in Table II. Although the results were superior when the skin was occluded, significant improvement was noted by many patients with the gel alone. Patients who responded to the gel also had a good response to 60% propylene glycol (60% P.G.),

Table III. Length of Treatment before Marked Improvement Was Noted[a]

Disease	Number of patients	Time (days)	
		60% P.G.	Keratolytic gel
Ichthyosis vulgaris	21	4-8	2-5
Sex-linked	6	4-7	2-4

[a]Occlusion was part of the treatment.

but only when occlusion was used. The time required for marked improvement of the skin was shorter when the keratolytic gel formulation was used compared to 60% P.G. (Table III). The gel with occlusion produced significant improvement of the hands within 1 week in 10 patients who showed dryness with extensive fissuring of the fingers. The improvement was manifested by healing of fissures and increased flexibility of the fingers. Some redness and peeling was noted in the hands, but this caused no symptoms. Six of the patients responded to 60% P.G., but the rate and degree of healing of fissures was not equal to the response obtained with the gel. The skin remained quite free of scales for 2–14 days with occlusion and 1–4 days without occlusion.

The results of the therapy with the gel in sex-linked ichthyosis were more dramatic (Fig. 2) than in the ichthyosis vulgaris, particularly when occlusion was used (Table II). All the patients showed complete or almost complete clearing when 60% P.G. was used under an occlusive plastic dressing, but improvement was much faster with the keratolytic gel (Table III). The length of the remission was similar to ichthyosis vulgaris.

Removal of scales in lamellar ichthyosis was achieved with the keratolytic gel (Fig. 3) but only when an occlusive plastic film was used (Table II). Less satisfactory results were oberved with 60% P.G. alone. Treatment with the gel had to be continued on a daily or alternate-day basis in order to maintain the effect.

The gel with and without occlusion gave inconsistent results in the management of 5 patients with epidermolytic hyperkeratosis.

Marked improvement of plantar hyperkeratosis within 2 weeks was achieved with the gel under occlusion (Fig. 4) in a variety of disorders: keratoderma climactericum (2); hyperkeratosis palmaris et plantaris

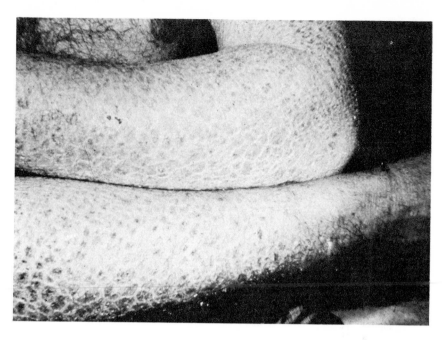

2a. Treatment of sex-linked ichthyosis with the keratolytic gel and a plastic dressing. A is before and B after treatment. The gel was used overnight for 4 days.

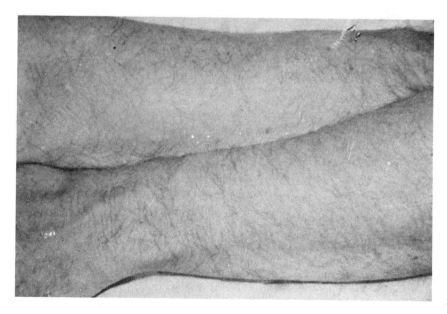

b.

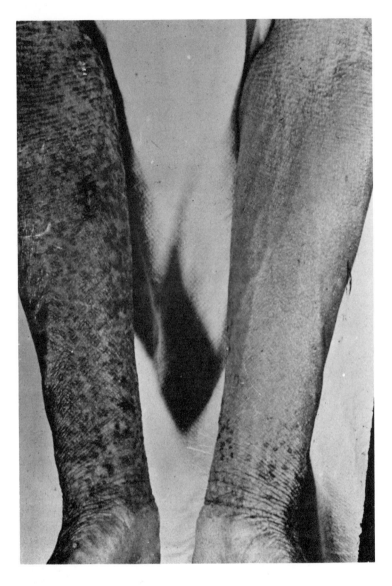

3   Treatment of lamellar ichthyosis with the keratolytic gel and a plastic dressing. The left side is untreated and the right side treated. The gel was used overnight for 1 week.

of Unna (2); pityriasis rubra pilaris (1); fungus infection (*T. rubrum*) (3); and psoriasis (6). In none of these patients did 60% PG give satisfactory improvement even under occlusion.

The keratolytic gel has also proved effective in a number of other disorders associated with hyperkeratosis. Keratosis pilaris responds rather promptly to nightly applications of the gel (Fig. 5). Lesions of the trunk respond well without occlusion while those of the extremities usually require a plastic dressing. The use of a lubricating ointment during the day will often lengthen the time of remission.

The roughened surface of actinically damaged skin may show a surprisingly dramatic response to the gel with or without occlusion. Very thick actinic keratoses, however, may require additional therapy, such as liquid nitrogen. Frequent use of an emollient cream will maintain the smooth appearance of the skin.

The so-called winter dryness which involves the hands, particularly the finger tips, and the lower legs may in reality represent a disorder of cell adherence. This condition will respond more rapidly and completely to a regimen involving the use of the keratolytic gel plus a lubricating ointment than to lubrication alone. A particularly effective regimen is the application of the gel, followed in 1 to 4 hours (depending on the response) by application of a lubricating agent. If occlusion is needed, the same dressing should be used for both preparations and left in place for a total of about 8 hours.

The keratolytic gel is also of value in treating certain fungal infections of the skin and is particularly effective in the fourth toe-web type and in tinea versicolor. Its use in these limited but recurrent fungal infections avoids contact with potentially sensitizing chemicals.

Ten patients with bilateral scaling and fissuring between the fourth and fifth toes were studied. Hyphae could be easily found on examination of the scales' and cultures were positive for *T. mentographytes* in 7 patients. The patients were instructed to apply the gel at night to the affected area on one foot and to wipe the treated area with a towel in the morning. At 1 week no maceration or fissuring was observed on the treated foot while the other side showed no improvement. The patient noted that improvement was detectable within 2 to 3 days on the treated side. Several patients described mild stinging in the fissures which lasted 5 to 10 minutes, but disappeared after the second application. Scrapings from the treated side were negative for hyphae and those from the other foot were positive. Both sides were then treated for a total of 1 month, when all patients were free of disease and scrapings were negative for fungi.

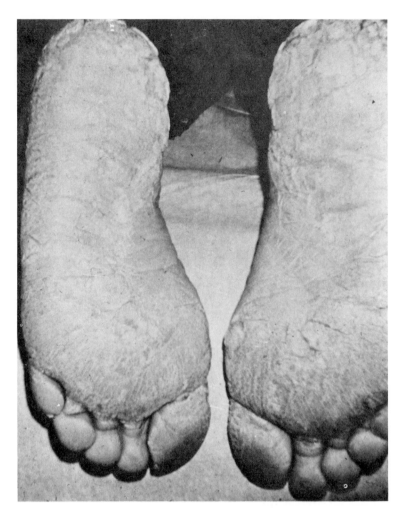

4 a. Before and after treatment of congenital hyperkeratosis of the soles with the keratolytic gel and a plastic dressing. The gel was used overnight for 2 weeks.

Ten patients with tinea versicolor, established by history, physical examination, and microscopic examination of scales were studied. All showed widespread involvement of the trunk, and scales showed numerous hyphae and spores. The patients were instructed to shower nightly and then apply the gel to the affected areas. At the end of 1

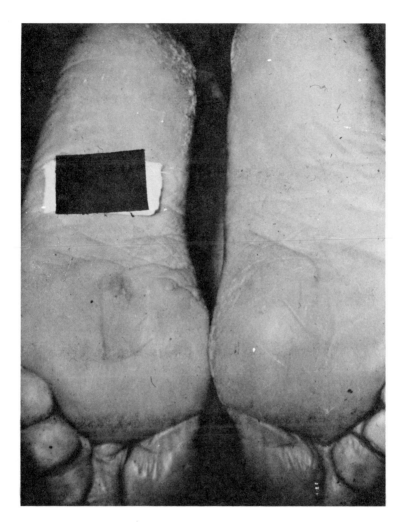

b.

week, scales were obtained from three lesions on each patient. In 3 patients some hyphae could be observed, but the number was clearly reduced. Therapy was continued for an additional week and scales obtained as before. In none of the patients could hyphae be found. Although some patients described dryness from the treatment, in only 2 was diffuse

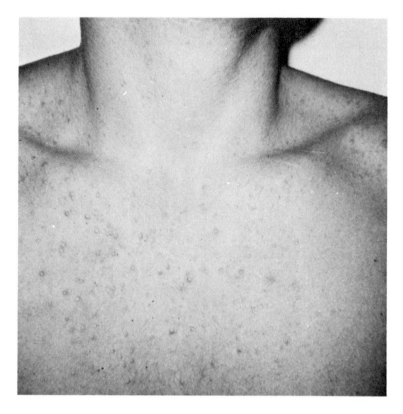

5 a. Treatment of keratosis pilaris with the keratolytic gel for 10 days without an occlusive dressing. A is before treatment and B after, showing marked improvement.

fine scaling visible and both were free of organisms at 1 week. Patients with hyperpigmented lesions noted that the dark color disappeared after several days of treatment.

In most of the disorders that have been discussed so far hyperkeratosis has been the principle manifestation, but there are numerous other diseases where this is only part of the problem. This is especially true of psoriasis and certain types of eczematous dermatitis. Not only is the thickened stratum corneum a problem on its own, but it can be a barrier to the penetration of other drugs such as corticosteroids. Keratolytic agents can therefore be used as an adjuvant by enhancing the

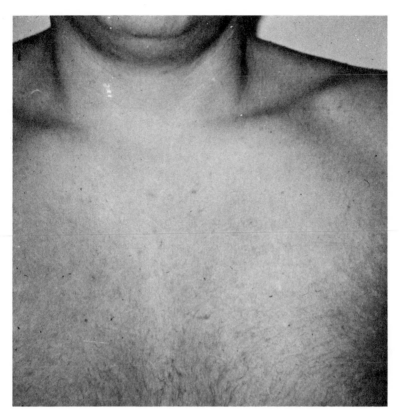

b.

penetration of other physical and chemical modalities.

This combination has been particularly effective in treating psoriasis and eczema of the palms associated with hyperkeratosis. The patients were instructed to soak their hands in tepid water in the evening, pat the skin dry, rub the keratolytic gel on one palm, and occlude with a plastic dressing for 2 to 4 hours. Following removal of the dressing, a fluorinated corticosteroid ointment was applied to both hands, and occlusion with plastic continued overnight.

On examination 2 weeks later, there was considerable improvement in the condition of both palms of all the patients. However, in each

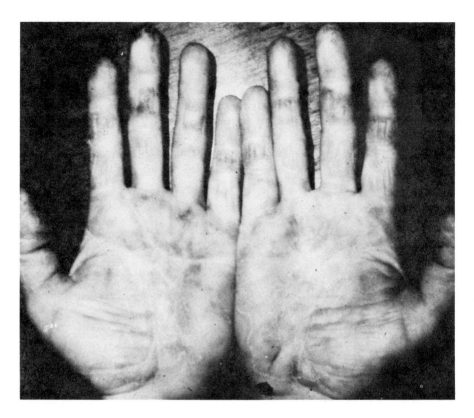

6 a. Treatment of Hyperkeratosis of the palms associated with an eczematous dermatitis. The hands were treated for 2 weeks overnight with a corticosteroid ointment (A) which resulted in significant improvement but left areas of hyperkeratosis (dark areas). The patient then used the keratolytic gel for 2 hours followed by the same corticosteroid overnight both under occlusion (B), which resulted in loss of the thickened stratum corneum within 2 weeks.

patient, the palm receiving the keratolytic gel showed no fissuring and little hyperkeratosis, while the other one had some fissures and consistently more hyperkeratosis (Figs. 6 and 7). The patients stated that both hands felt improved, but some painful fissuring was present on the hand that had not been treated with the gel.

As an extension of this study, we investigated the use of the ker-

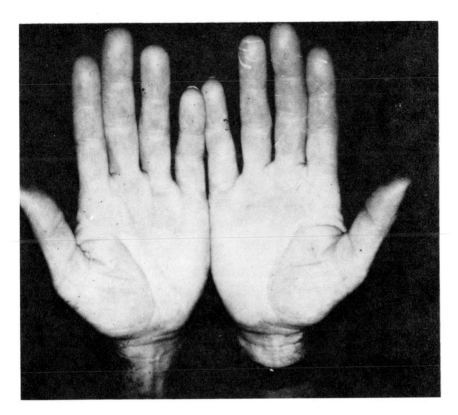

b.

atolytic gel and corticosteroid sequential treatment in more generalized psoriasis. The length of treatment with the keratolytic gel was 1 to 4 hours depending on the thickness of the lesions. Plastic exercise suits were used for occlusion since they save a considerable amount of time. When patients were studied by paired comparison the combination treatment was clearly superior to the steroid alone and it resulted in almost complete clearing in 2 weeks. This regimen was also successful for the scalp but a steroid preparation in propylene glycol was used.

An additional use of the keratolytic agents was in combination with ultraviolet light (UVL). The abnormal and thickened stratum corneum

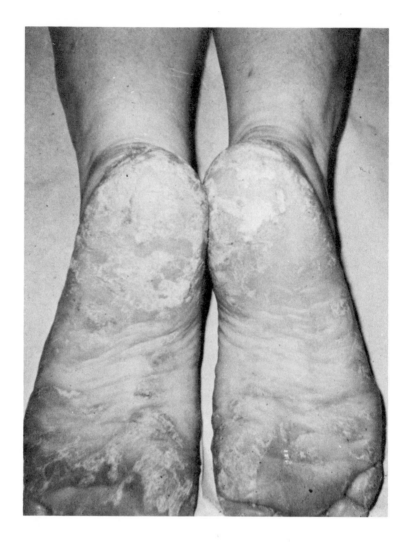

7 a. Treatment of psoriasis of the soles. The feet were treated for 2 weeks overnight with a corticosteroid ointment (A) which resulted in some improvement. The patient then used the keratolytic gel for 2 hours followed by the same corticosteroid ointment overnight both under occlusion (B), which resulted in a striking improvement.

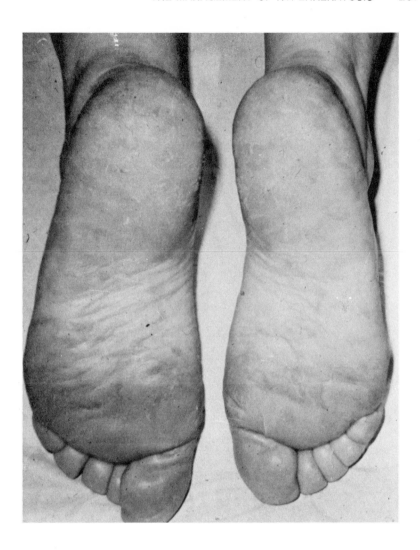

b.

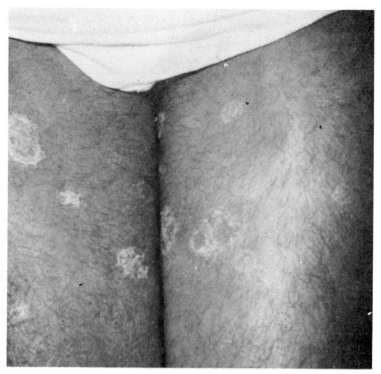

8   The effect of the keratolytic gel on increasing the response of the skin to ultraviolet light (UVB). The right leg was treated with the gel under a plastic dressing nightly for 4 days and the patient was then given a dose of UVB calculated to be a minimal erythema dose for the normal skin. The right leg (darker) was much redder at 24 hours.

Table IV. Conditions Successfully Treated with Keratolytic gel

Ichthyosis
Seborrheic dermatitis
Psoriasis
Chronic eczematous dermatitis
Dry (winter) skin
Sun-damaged skin
Pityriasis Rubra Pilaris
Tinea pedis
Tinea versicolor
Hyperkeratosis of palms and soles
Keratosis pilaris
Acne
Warts
Actinic Keratoses

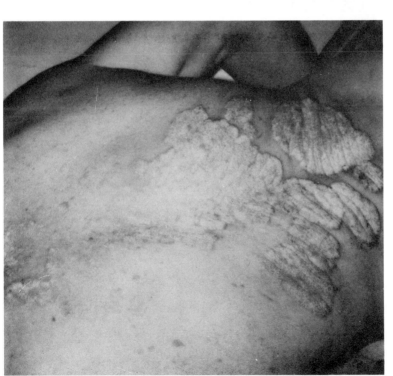

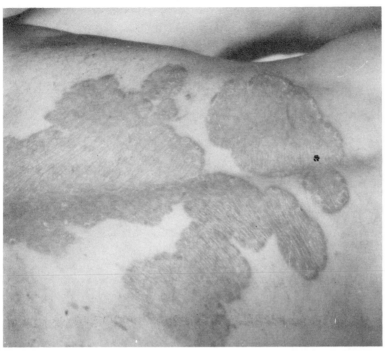

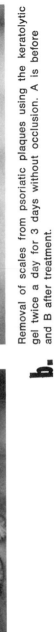

b. Removal of scales from psoriatic plaques using the keratolytic gel twice a day for 3 days without occlusion. A is before and B after treatment.

9 a.

can absorb and scatter ultraviolet light and reduce the amount of energy penetrating into the viable layers of the epidermis. Removal of this hyperkeratotic tissue would allow more penetration of ultraviolet light and greater inhibition of epidermal cell metabolism. This even occurs in normal epidermis where an increased erythema response to UVL is observed following treatment with keratolytic gel for several days (Fig. 8). A consistent finding during treatment with UVL is that certain lesions particularly those on the extremities are more resistant to treatment. This is seen when both UVA and UVB are used. By using the keratolytic gel daily, most effectively with occlusion for 2–4 hours, these resistant plaques are seen to respond more rapidly.

SUMMARY

The keratolytic gel is an effective therapeutic modality for treating a variety of disorders associated with hyperkeratosis. The preparation will remove thickened stratum corneum but has no direct effect on inflammatory disorders associated with them. It can be used, however, very successfully in combination with other modalities. In Table IV is a list of conditions, which have been treated with considerable improvement.
Certain guidelines should be followed in using the keratolytic preparation: (1) Hydration of the skin before use of the gel increases its effectiveness and reduces the chance of irritation. When treating the scalp the gel is applied to the skin and then the hair is lightly moistened with water. (2) Open treatment should be tried first and this may be enhanced by applying a lubricant several hours after using the gel and repeating this once or twice a day (Fig. 9). (3) Before occluding the skin the gel should be allowed to dry so that most of the alcohol will volatilize. (4) The length of occlusive treatment should be adjusted to the response of the patient; too much causes irritation and with too little, there is no response. (5) Irrespective of how the gel is used, a lubricant should be applied at least once a day for maximum effectiveness.

ACKNOWLEDGMENT

Research Supported by N.I.H. Grant AM 06838.

REFERENCES

1. G.F. Odland and T.H. Reed, Epidermis, in "Uultrastructure of Normal and Abnormal Skin," (A.S. Zelickson ed.), pp. 54–75. Lea & Febiger, Philadelphia, 1967.
2. E. Christophers, H.H. Wolf, and E.B. Lawrence, The formation of epidermal cell columns, J. Invest. Dermatol. 62, 555–559 (1974).
3. A.G. Matoltsy, "Biology of the Skin and Hair Growth" (A.G. Lyne and B.F. Short, eds.), p. 291. Elsevier, Amsterdam, 1965.
4. K.M. Rudall, The proteins of the mammalian epidermis, in "Advances in Protein Chemistry, M.L. Anson, K. Bailey, and J.T. Edsall, pp, 253–290. Academic Press, Inc., New York, 1952.
5. H.P. Baden, L.A. Goldsmith, and B. Fleming, Polypeptide composition of epidermal prekeratin. Biochim. Biophys. Acta 317, 303–311 (1973).
6. H.P. Baden and L. Bonar, The α fibrous proteins of epidermis, J. Invest. Dermatol. 51, 478–483 (1968).
7. H.P. Baden and L.A. Goldsmith, Changes in the α fibrous protein during epidermal keratinization. Acta Dermatovener 51, 321–326 (1971).
8. H.P. Baden, L.A. Goldsmith, and B. Fleming. Comparative study of the physicochemical properties of human keratinized tissues, Biochim. Biophys. Acta 322, 269–278 (1973).
9. L.A. Sirback, R.H. Gray, and I.A. Bernstein, Localization of the histidine-rich peptide in keratohyalin: A morphologic and macromolecular marker in epidermal differentiation, J. Invest. Dermatol. 62, 394–405 (1974).
10. A.G. Matoltsy, R.M. Looker, and M.N. Matoltsy, Demonstration of cystine-containing protein in keratohyalin granules of the epidermis. J. Invest. Dermatol. 62, 406–410 (1974).
11. L.A. Goldsmith and H.P. Baden, Uniquely oriented epidermal lipid, Nature (London) 225, 1052–1053 (1970).
12. A.S. Breathnack, Development of dermal elements, in "An Atlas of Ultrastructure of Human Skin," p. 79. J. & A. Churchill, London, 1971.
13. P. Frisch, K. Wolff, and H. Honigsmann, Glycocalyx of epidermal cells in vitro: demonstration and enzymatic removal, J. Invest. Dermatol. 64, 30–37 (1975).
14. H.H. Roenigk, H.I. Maibach, and G.D. Weinstein, Use of methotrexate in psoriasis, Arch, Dermat. 105, 363–365 (1972).
15. I.H. Blank, Further observations on factors which influence the water content of the stratum corneum, J. Invest. Dermatol. 21, 259–269 (1954).
16. M.R. Lerner and A.B. Lerner, "Dermatologic Medications," The Year Book Publishers, Inc., Chicago, Illinois, 1960.

17. L.A. Goldsmith and H.P. Baden, Propylene glycol with occlusion in ichthyosis. *JAMA* 220, 579–580 (1972).
18. H.P. Baden and J.C. Alper, A keratolytic gel containing salicylic acid in propylene glycol. *J. Invest. Dermatol.* 61, 330–333 (1973).
19. H.P. Baden, Treatment of hyperkeratotic dermatitis of the palms. *Arch. Dermatol.* 110, 737–738 (1974).

21

Topical Insect Repellents: Volatility Modifications

HOWARD I. MAIBACH
A. A. KHAN

Repellents are chemicals which result in the insects making oriented movements away from their source (1). They have several advantages over other methods of protection. They do not kill insects; hence, genetic selection of resistant insects does not take place. They are not sprayed, like insecticides, on vast areas; hence, environmental pollution does not occur. They do not need a vast organization and elaborate equipment for application but are handy and can be carried in a pocket.

Considering the above advantages, repellents should be an ideal solution for protection against insect bites. Their limitations are considerable; they are ineffective over long periods of time with one application and must be applied every few hours depending on the temperature, humidity, wind speed (2), the density of the blood feeding species (3) (Table I), and the variety of the blood feeding insect fauna (4). They must be applied on all exposed skin areas, and even on clothes, when in areas heavily infested with mosquitoes. They feel oily, irritate mucous membrane, stain clothes and dissolve plastics, are easily rubbed off or washed off, and fail against some species.

243

Table I. Mean Protection Time of Repellents Tested Against Different
Densities of *aedes aegypti* Females in a Cage[a]

Repellent (0.16 mg/cm^2)	Density/Cage		
	100	500	2,000
Triethylene glycol monohexyl ether	11.5	9.7	6.6
1,1'-carboxyl-*bis*-hexamethyleneimine	9.8	7.6	2.5
Deet	5.1	4.3	3.4

[a]Each figure is a mean of 7 replicates.

MODE OF ACTION

Most repellents act through vapor from a distance. Volatility of a compound, therefore, is critical. More volatile repellents drive away insects from a great distance but are quickly lost; consequently the protection period is short. Less volatile repellents or solids protect at a shorter distance or only on contact. These may last longer but their effectiveness may be considerably decreased for lack of enough vapor concentration on the applied surface.

The effectiveness of a repellent also depends on its intrinsic repellency. Compounds with high intrinsic repellency repel at low vapor concentration and will last longer. The minimum effective dose (MED), i.e., the dose below which a repellent is ineffective, varies from repellent to repellent (Table II). Among compounds of similar boiling point, one with higher intrinsic repellency will prove the better repellent.

MINIMIZING LOSS OF REPELLENT THROUGH EVAPORATION

The principal sources of repellent loss are evaporation, abrasion from the skin surface, and percutaneous absorption (5). Several workers attempted to minimize loss through evaporation by formulating repellents with special vehicles. Formulations containing zinc oxide were more effective than pure repellent at the same dilution but not better than full strength repellent (5).

Table II. Mean Protection Time of Repellents Applied at 0.16 mg/cm^2 and Respective Minimum Effective Dose (MED)

			Repellents				
	Deet		**Triethylene glycol mono- hexyl either**		**Hexamethylene butanesulf- onamide**	**1,1'-carboxyl-*bis*- (hexamethyl eneimine**	
Protection MED time (hour)/ mg/cm^2	4.2	0.1	6.5	0.2	10.0 0.1	9.2	0.2
No. of replicates	8	7	12	7	12 5	9	5

In the perfume industry fixatives are commonly used. Most fragrances are volatile and are rapidly lost. To make perfumes last longer fixatives are added. A fixative is a relatively less volatile constituent which depresses the volatility of the other components. Fixatives include musks, civit, ambergris, etc. We mixed 7 synthetic musks combined in 3 different ratios with 4 insect repellents. The formulations were tested by applying a measured quantity with a fine pipette on a 5- × 25-cm marked area on the human forearm and exposing the treated area to 250–300 female *Aedes aegypti* (L.) in a 1 cu ft cage for 3 minutes. The untreated area of the forearm and the hand were wrapped in plastic to prevent biting. The mosquitoes had no previous blood meal and were fed 5% sugar water only. The 3-minute exposure to mosquitoes was repeated every 30 minutes until two bites were obtained. The duration from application to two bites was termed protection time. Four fixatives gave increased protection with diethyltoluamide (deet) depending on formulation ratios (6) (Table III). These were musk Tibetene®, ambrette, givambrol, and musk xylol. None proved effective with dimethylphthalate, ethyl hexanediol, or Indalone®.

We extended the study to vanillin (4-hydroxy-3-methoxy-benzaldehyde) as a prolongator of insect repellents. Seven repellents were tested combined with vanillin in four different ratios. Vanillin was effective with all. The increase in protection time with different ratios of vanillin

Table III. Percent Increase in Protection Time Against Mosquito Bites
Obtained with Deet on Formulation with Musks in Different Ratios

Musks	Formulation (mg/cm^2) repellent/musk	Increase (%)
Tibetene®	0.16 + 0.16	29
	0.16 + 0.32	47
	0.16 + 0.48	88
	0.32 + 0.16	24
	0.32 + 0.32	12
	0.32 + 0.48	18
Ambrette	0.16 + 0.16	33
	0.32 + 0.32	25
	0.32 + 0.48	16
Givambrol	0.32 + 0.16	37
	0.32 + 0.32	43
Musk xylol	0.32 + 0.16	30

to repellents was significant only with deet. In most cases the increase in protection time was in excess of 100% (7) (Table IV).

IMPROVING WATER-WASH RESISTANCE OF REPELLENTS

Repellents are lost in minutes on coming in contact with water as may occur in fishing or on beaches. The amount of deet protecting dry skin for several hours loses effectiveness within 2 minutes when exposed to free flowing water. Thus in rain or on wading through water a fresh application of the repellent is needed almost immediately. To minimize this loss it is necessary to incorporate the repellent in the matrix of a hydrophobic vehicle. We employed co-polypers of hydroxy-vinyl chloride-acetate for this. The polymers were tested with several repellents with significant improvement in water washability (Table V). Cosmetic acceptability was inadequate.

REPELLENTS IMPREGNATED ON NETTING

Repellents applied to the skin are lost through evaporation, abrasion, and excretion, mandating repeated application. On netting, they last

Table IV. Percent Increase in Protection Time Against Mosquito Bites Obtained with Different Repellents Mixed with Vanillin in Different Ratios

Repellent	Formulation (mg/cm^2) repellent/musk	Increase (%)
Deet	0.16 + 0.16	95
	0.16 + 0.32	142
	0.26 + 0.48	178
Ethyl hexanediol	0.16 + 0.16	75
	0.16 + 0.32	90
	0.16 + 0.48	105
Dimethyl phthalate	0.16 + 0.16	180
	0.16 + 0.32	180
	0.16 + 0.48	140
Indalone®	0.16 + 0.16	87
	0.16 + 0.32	120
	0.16 + 0.48	133
Triethylene glycol monohexyl ether	0.16 + 0.08	94
	0.16 + 0.16	103
	0.16 + 0.32	112
Triethylene glycol monoheptyl ether	0.16 + 0.08	80
	0.16 + 0.16	63
	0.16 + 0.32	127
Triethylene glycol ethyl hexyl ether	0.16 + 0.08	153
	0.16 + 0.16	134
	0.16 + 0.32	165

much longer. Compounds that are potent repellents but cannot be used on skin because they are lost too quickly through absorption can be used impregnated on netting to be worn over clothing as a jacket. Repellent-treated netting for protection against biting insects can be used as a bed net, head net, or net to cover windows, etc. Repellent-treated net jackets may be worn on top of a shirt to protect biting through clothing or under hot and humid conditions can be worn without underclothing, i.e., as a shirt, next to the skin (8).

We used wide mesh (3/inches) knotted cotton netting for evaluating repellents. This has the advantage of giving good ventilation and im-

Table V. Increase in Wash Resistance of Repellents with the
Addition of Polymers[a)b]

Repellent	Time (minutes) to 2 bites without polymer	Time (minutes) to 2 bites with polymers
Triethylene glycol monohexyl ether	0.7	15
Ethyl hexanediol	1.4	11
Deet	1.7	19
Indalone®	1.9	8
Hexamethylene butane sulfonamide	2.0	10
Dimethyl phthalate	2.2	6

[a]Repellent applied at 1.6 mg/cm^2 + polymer at 6.4 mg/cm^2.
[b]Water-flow was at 6 liters/minute at 30°C.

proved visibility and hearing (9). One gram of netting was soaked in
0.25 gm of repellent. It was attached to the bottom of a glass cylinder
50-cm high and 9-cm in diameter. Twenty mosquitoes (*A. aegypti*) previously fed on sugar water only were placed in the glass cylinder. The
top of the cylinder was covered with netting. The human palm or the
forearm was exposed under the netting abutted against it for 3 minutes.
This was repeated twice a week until two bites were obtained. The
netting was then discarded.

Results (Table VI) show that deet lost effectiveness sooner than
the three other repellents. The triethylene glycol ether, the carboxamide,
and the sulfonamide proved superior to deet on netting.

CONCLUSIONS

Ten to twenty thousand compounds have been screened for use as
topical repellents (10). However, no repellent is entirely satisfactory.
Mixing additives with deet and other known repellents increases their
protection time. This is a useful lead and needs development. Polymers,
if combined with repellents enhance their abrasion resistance and water
wash resistance. The problem of cosmetic acceptability requires resolution.

Table VI. Time in Days from Impregnation to Breakdown of Repellents on Wide-Mesh Netting When Tested Against *Aedes aegypti* on Human Skin[a]

Deet	Triethylene glycol monohexyl ether (C_8 straight chain compound)	1,1-carboxyl-*bis*- (hexamethylene-imine)	Hexamethyleneimine butane sulfonamide
68	151 +	78	151 +

[a]One gm of net was soaked in 0.25g of repellent.

Deet-treated net parkas and trousers are available commercially but are rather expensive and not sufficiently publicized. It is claimed that they remain effective for about 3 months. Protective clothing of this kind could become popular if made cheaper and if facilities for recharging the clothing are easily available.

There is a need for continued investigation into the mode of action of insect repellents, synthesis and screening of new compounds for repellent action, study of physiological and morphological receptor mechanisms in hematophagous insects, and study of the host seeking behavior of blood feeders and the attractive principle(s) emanated by the host. If enough basic and necessary information in all these areas can be developed, it is possible, even probable, that a systemic insect repellent may be available.

REFERENCES

1. V.G. Dethier, et al., The designation of chemicals in terms of the response they elicit from insects. *J. Econ. Entomol.* 53, 134–136 (1960).
2. A.A. Khan, et al., A study of insect repellents. 2. Effect of temperature on protection time. *J. Econ. Entomol.* 66, 437–438 (1973).
3. A.A. Khan, et al., insect repellents: Effect of mosquito and repellent related factors on protection time. *J. Econ. Entomol.* 68, 43–45 (1975).
4. I.H. Gilbert, et al., Repellents against mosquitoes in Thailand. *J. Econ. Entomol.* 63, 1207–1209 (1970).
5. C.N. Smith, Repellents for anopheline mosquitoes. *Misc. Publ. Ent. Soc. Amer.* 7, 99:115 (1970).
6. A.A. Khan, et al., Addition of perfume fixatives to mosquito repellents to increase protection time. *Mosquito News* 35, 23–26 (1975).
7. A.A. Khan, et al., Addition of vanillin to mosquito repellents to increase

protection time. *Mosquito News* 35, 223–225 (1975).

8. E.P. Catts, Deet-impregnated net shirt repels biting flies. *J. Econ. Entomol.* 61, 1765 (1968).

9. R.H. Grothaus, et al., An innovation in mosquito-borne disease protection. *Military Med.* 137, 181–184 (1972).

10. W.V. King, Chemicals evaluated as insecticides and repellents at Orlando, Florida. *USDA Agr. Handbook* 69, 397 pp. (1954).

Index

vaginal infection, and silver sulfadiazine, 52
Valisone. *See* betamethasone valerate
vanillin, as insect-repellent fixative, 245-246, *247*
vascular surgery, and silver sulfadiazine, 51-52
vasoconstriction assay, 107
    principles of, 106
vehicles
    for alpha-hydroxy acid (and related compounds), 212
    in dermatopharmacological evaluation, 138-139
    importance of, 197-198
    for insect repellents, 246
    and stratum corneum breakdown, 223
venereal disease, and silver sulfadiazine, 52
vitamin A acid, and keratinization, 212

warts, transfer factor for, 70-73
water, in intracellular cementing process, 223
watt, and photochemotherapy, 195
winter dryness, keratolytic gel and, 229

xenografts, 49

zinc oxide, in insect repellents, 244
zinc sulfadiazine, 49
    mode of action of, 51
    and psoriasis, 52
zinc therapy, 44